Color Atlas of

AIDS

and HIV Disease

Second Edition

Charles F. Farthing, MB, ChB, MRCP, FRACP

Research Registrar in AIDS,
St. Stephen's Hospital, London

Simon E. Brown, FIMBI, ABIPP, ARPS

Chief Photographer,
formerly at Charing Cross & Westminster Medical School, London

Richard C.D. Staughton, MA (Cantab), FRCP

Consultant Physician to the Skin Departments
Westminster and St. Stephen's Hospitals, London

Contributing authors to first edition:

Jeffrey J. Cream, BSc (Hons), MD, FRCP
Consultant Dermatologist,
Charing Cross Hospital, London

Mark Mühlemann, BSc (Hons), MB, BS, MRCP
formerly Senior Registrar,
Department of Dermatology,
Charing Cross Hospital, London

Year Book Medical Publishers, Inc

Copyright © C.F. Farthing, S.E. Brown, R.C.D. Staughton, 1988

This book is copyrighted in England and distributed
in Continental North America, Hawaii and Puerto Rico
by Year Book Medical Publishers, Inc., 200 North
LaSalle Street, Chicago, Illinois 60601, USA, by
arrangement with Wolfe Medical Publications Ltd.
Printed by W.S. Cowell Ltd, Ipswich, England

Library of Congress Cataloging-in-Publication Data

Color atlas of AIDS/Charles F. Farthing...(et al.). –
2nd ed. p. cm.
   Rev. ed. of: A Colour atlas of AIDS (acquired
immunodeficiency syndrome). 1986.
   Includes index.
   ISBN 0-8151-3246-8
   1. AIDS (Disease) – Atlases. I. Farthing, Charles F.
   (DNLM: 1. Acquired Immunodeficiency Syndrome –
   atlases. WD 308 C719)
RC607.A26C65 1988
616.97′92 – dc19
DNLM/DLC
for Library of Congress

Contents

To our patients and colleagues

Acknowledgements

We wish to thank our colleagues for all their encouragement and advice in the production of this atlas.

Histopathology: Dr. A. C. Branfoot, Dr. J. N. Harcourt-Webster, Professor Kristin Henry.

Medical microbiology: Dr. R. E. Evans, Miss Jenny Midgely, Dr. D. C. Shanson.

Cytology: Dr. O. A. N. Husain.

And our clinical colleagues Dr. N. G. Gazzard, Dr. A. G. Lawrence, Dr. R. H. Phillips, Dr. J. Collins, and Professor C. Wastell.

Our thanks also to Dr. Kwesi Tsiquaye (London School of Hygiene) and R. Jonathan Webet (National Cancer Institute) for providing material.

We would like to pay tribute to the nursing, technical and administrative staff of our hospitals, for their devoted care and attention to our patients.

Our special thanks go to Miss Kath Meikle for typing the text.

We acknowledge the following for photographs:
E.M. Department, London School of Hygiene
Professor Kristin Henry
Professor A. Guz
A. Boyleston
I. Murray-Lyon
P. G. Elliott
Miss G. Midgely
A. G. Lawrence

The illustrations in Appendix B, AIDS in Africa, are the copyright of M. Rolfe.

Part 1 The AIDS epidemic

Section 1: Epidemiology

The Acquired Immunodeficiency Syndrome (AIDS) was first recognised in Los Angeles and New York in 1981 with an extraordinary outbreak of *Pneumocystis carinii* pneumonia and Kaposi's sarcoma in previously fit young men. Before this date in the USA both conditions had been very rare. Previously, *Pneumocystis carinii* pneumonia had been confined to those immunocompromised by age, known malignant disease or immunosuppressive therapy. Kaposi's sarcoma had been seen usually in those of Jewish, Mediterranean and African extraction. The new cases were found to be occurring in special risk groups and in people indulging in certain risk practices, suggesting that a single infection with a blood- and semen-borne virus, like the hepatitis B virus, might be responsible.

Table 1

Risk groups and practices	
Homosexual intercourse	72%
Intravenous drug use	17%
Haitian	4%
Haemophiliacs	1%
Blood transfusion recipients	1%
Heterosexual partners	1%
Unclassified	4%

(CDC figures for USA 1982)

Soon, other opportunistic infections were described in the same risk groups:

Table 2

Protozoa	*Virus*	
Pneumocystis carinii	Cytomegalovirus	
Toxoplasma gondii	Herpes simplex	(The herpes group)
Cryptosporidia	Herpes zoster	
	Epstein-Barr	
Fungi	Bacteria	
Candida albicans	Atypical mycobacteria	
Cryptococcus neoformans		

The marked bias towards protozoal, fungal and viral organisms suggested a defect of cell mediated immunity. The relative absence of bacterial sepsis suggested that humoral (antibody mediated) immunity was left relatively intact.

AIDS was therefore defined in 1982 as Kaposi's sarcoma in a person under 60 years of age or an opportunistic infection suggestive of a *defect in cell mediated immunity* occurring in a person with *no known cause* for a diminished resistance to the particular disease with which they presented. The definition has subsequently been changed several times in light of recent discoveries (see Section 4 for the current definition).

The numbers of cases of AIDS were noted to rise steadily and dramatically in each country in which the epidemic occurred. At any one point in time about half the cases of AIDS reported have died.

Cumulative totals, including deaths, 1986 and 1987

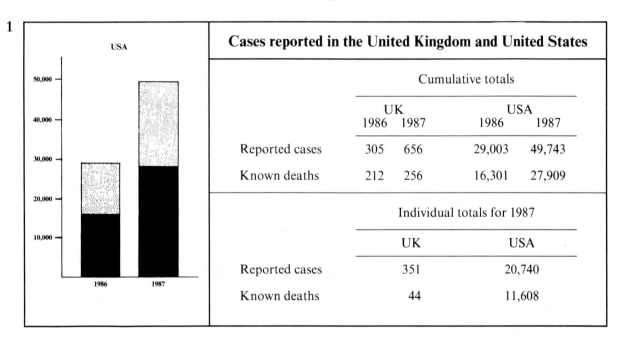

Cases reported in the United Kingdom and United States

	Cumulative totals			
	UK 1986	UK 1987	USA 1986	USA 1987
Reported cases	305	656	29,003	49,743
Known deaths	212	256	16,301	27,909

	Individual totals for 1987	
	UK	USA
Reported cases	351	20,740
Known deaths	44	11,608

1   The graph shows the incidence of AIDS in the United States. The cumulative totals include known deaths which are represented by the solidly shaded areas. The table shows the number of cases reported in the United Kingdom and the United States.

Section 2: Immunology

Immunological investigation of patients with AIDS revealed the defect in cell mediated immunity that the pattern of opportunistic infections suggested. Three particular abnormalities on immune function testing were found to be occurring together in an unusual and distinctive combination that has come to be known as the AIDS triad:

1. Decreased numbers of helper T (or CD4 positive) lymphocytes (often leading to a decreased T-helper/T-suppressor ratio and to an absolute lymphopenia).

2. Hypergammaglobulinaemia (a polyclonal rise in IgG).

3. Impaired response to recall antigens on skin testing (i.e. impaired delayed type hypersensitivity "DTH").

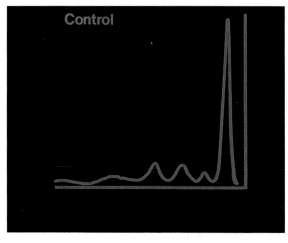

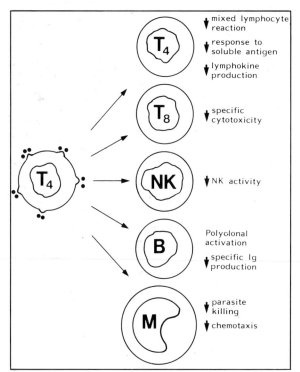

2 **The T-helper lymphocyte** has been described as the conductor of the immunological orchestra and certainly it influences the function of many other cells in the immune system, including B lymphocyte and macrophage function as shown. Most defects in immune function described in AIDS can be explained by a decrease in T-helper lymphocyte function.

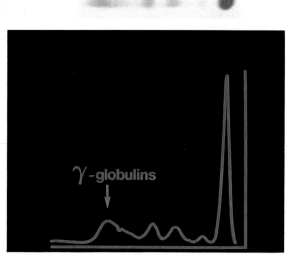

3 Protein electrophoretic strip of serum in a patient with AIDS showing a polyclonal rise in gammaglobulins.

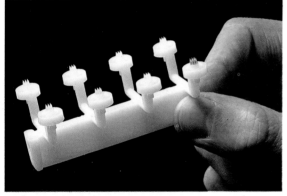

4 **A multiple applicator** for delayed-type hypersensitivity skin testing, tests for trichophyton, proteus, streptococcus, tuberculin, candida, diphtheria, tetanus and a control.

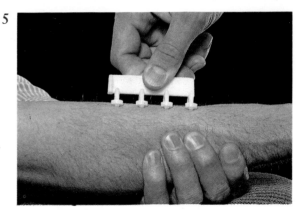

5 **Application to forearm.**

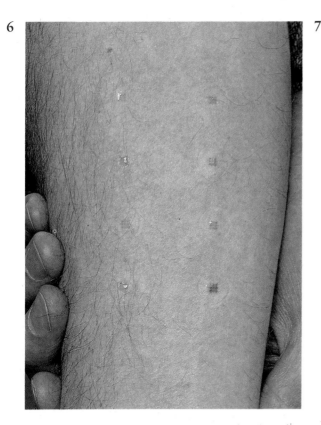

6 Forearm showing imprint immediately after application.

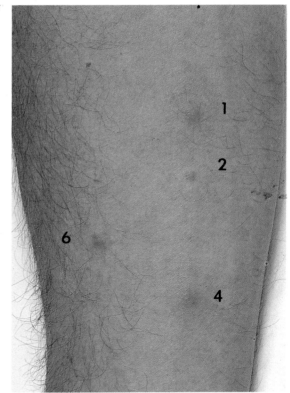

7 Same forearm showing normal response to tetanus, diphtheria, tuberculin and *Candida* at 48 hours. A lesser response is usually seen in patients with AIDS.

Section 3: Virology

In 1983 Barre-Sinoussi and colleagues in Paris isolated a retrovirus from a patient with lymphadenopathy. They named the virus Lymphadenopathy Associated Virus (LAV). In 1984 Gallo and colleagues in the USA isolated a retrovirus they termed Human T cell Lymphotropic Virus type III (HTLV III) from several patients with AIDS. These two isolates have subsequently been found to be identical, and are now recognised to be the cause of AIDS. The virus is now termed the Human Immunodeficiency Virus (HIV).

8

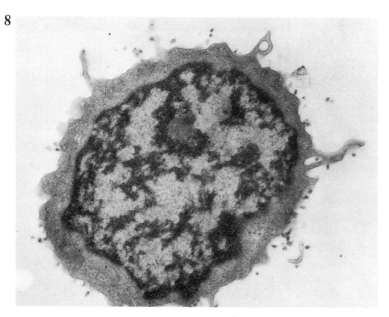

8 A malignant T-lymphocyte growing in cell culture showing budding of HIV virions from the cell surface. HIV is difficult to maintain in cell culture unless rapidly growing malignant T-cells are used. Ordinary T-lymphocyte cell cultures are rapidly killed off by HIV.

9

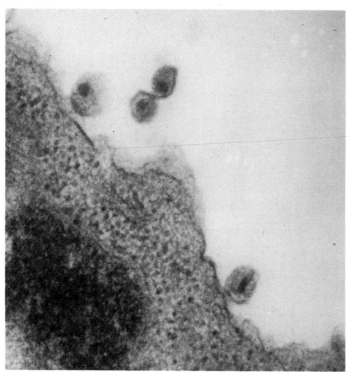

9 Close-up of HIV virions budding from the cell surface. The conical protein core of the virus can be seen both in longitudinal and cross-section, surrounded by a glycoprotein outer membrane.

Retroviruses are RNA viruses, their name referring to the fact that RNA transcription proceeds in a reverse direction (RNA to DNA) before the viral genome can be incorporated into the host genome and viral replication commence. This essential retrograde step is dependent upon the presence of a viral enzyme called reverse transcriptase. Pharmacological inhibition of this enzyme inhibits replication of HIV. Zidovudine is an inhibitor of reverse transcriptase.

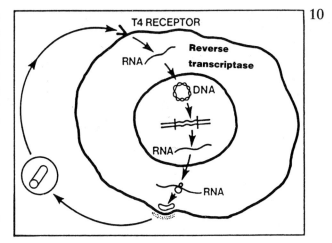

10 Diagrammatic representation of retrovirus replication.

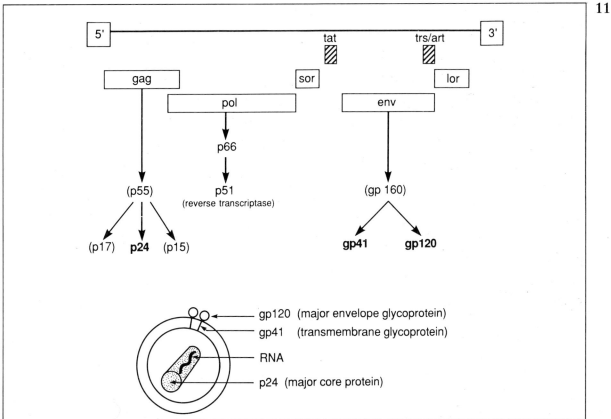

11 Schematic representation of the genome of HIV. Three principal genes code for the group associated antigen (gag), the reverse transcriptase or polymerase (pol), and the envelope glycoproteins (env). The principal core protein is of molecular weight 24,000 (p24). The principal envelope glycoproteins are of molecular weight 41,000 and 120,000 (gp41 and gp120). Precursor proteins of molecular weight 55,000 and 160,000 (p55 and gp160) are formed in infected cells, but are not present in intact virus particles. The two small genes tat and trs/art encode for proteins which are believed to be essential for regulating virus assembly within cells. It is thought that a drug to block transcription of the tat gene or to inhibit the product of its transcription may be another effective way of halting HIV replication. The genes sor and lor (short and long open reading frames) encode for proteins with functional roles which are yet to be determined.

Section 4: The definition of AIDS

AIDS is defined as *a disease* indicative of a defect in cell mediated immunity occurring in a person with no known cause for immunodeficiency *other than the presence of HIV*.

The diseases accepted as indicating a defect in cell mediated immunity are strictly listed by CDC (Center for Disease Control, Atlanta, Georgia). Some may be presumptively diagnosed, others must be definitely diagnosed. Some must have been causing illness in the patient for longer than one month. For some the presence of HIV infection must be proven, for others not.

The major diseases that are considered to indicate a defect in cell mediated immunity and thus define a person as having AIDS are:

Protozoal:

Pneumocystis carinii pneumonia (PCP)
Toxoplasmosis of the brain
Cryptosporidiosis with diarrhoea > one month.

Fungal:

Candidiasis – oesophageal, tracheal, bronchial or pulmonary (oral thrush alone is insufficient for a diagnosis of AIDS)
Cryptococcus – meningitis (or other extrapulmonary site).

Viral:

Cytomegalovirus (CMV) – retinitis, pneumonitis, colitis or encephalitis

Herpes simplex – mucocutaneous disease > one month

Progressive multifocal leucoencephalopathy (PML).

Bacterial:

Mycobacterium avium intracellulare (MAI) or *M. kansasii* – disseminated

M. tuberculosis (if extrapulmonary and not confined only to lymph glands in a patient who is HIV antibody positive)

Recurrent non typhoid salmonella septicaemia (if patient HIV antibody positive).

Tumours

Kaposi's sarcoma — any age if patient HIV antibody positive (<60 if HIV status unknown).
Primary CNS lymphoma

Non-Hodgkin's lymphoma of B cell type (only if patient HIV antibody positive).

Others

HIV encephalopathy (HIV brain and spinal cord disease/AIDS dementia complex – if patient HIV antibody positive)

HIV wasting syndrome ("slim disease") – if patient HIV antibody positive

Lymphoid interstitial pneumonitis (LIP) in child <13 years of age.

For the full CDC definition of AIDS see Appendix A.

Section 5: The antibody response to HIV

The vast majority of patients infected with HIV can be shown to have circulating antibodies to HIV viral proteins. However, a small number of patients have been demonstrated to be infected with virus, by virus isolation and antigen assay techniques, and yet be seronegative for antibodies. Thus, if clinical signs and symptoms suggestive of HIV disease are present but the antibody test is negative, a clinician should not necessarily dismiss the diagnosis.

It is now generally believed that any patient seropositive for HIV antibodies remains infected and infectious for life. This is in contradistinction to hepatitis B where the presence of antibodies means that the patient is no longer infectious. (HIV may be isolated from greater than 80% of HIV antibody positive individuals up to six years after infection, and related animal retroviruses consistently result in persisting infection.)

Antibodies for HIV usually appear in the blood some five to 12 weeks after infection, antibody to the transmembrane glycoprotein gp41 usually being detectable prior to the development of antibody to the principal core protein p24 (see **12**).

HIV antigen can now be measured by an ELISA technique. Its estimation, however, is not generally as useful a test for screening for the presence of HIV as the HIV antibody test. Antigen is detectable early in the disease (see **12**) when a 'seroconversion illness' may be apparent clinically (see Section 9) and then, as antibodies appear in the serum, it usually becomes undetectable. Much later in the course of the illness and often as HIV disease is starting to become symptomatic with the development of ARC or AIDS, the anti p24 antibody titre may fall and HIV antigen again become detectable in the serum (see **12**).

The HIV antigen test is therefore useful for detecting the presence of early infection prior to seroconversion and in later disease as a marker of disease progression. A persistently positive antigen test is generally considered to indicate a poor prognosis. However, it should be noted that some patients persistently positive for HIV antigen for some years are not rapidly deteriorating and some who do poorly are negative for HIV antigen.

12

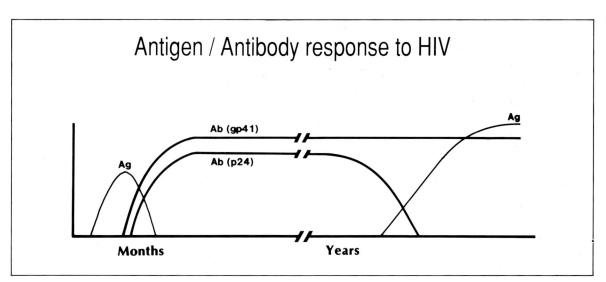

12 **Schematic representation of the antigen/antibody response to HIV.** Antigen appears in the blood usually within a few weeks. First antibody to the HIV viral coat glycoprotein gp41 and then antibody to the core protein p24 appear in the serum. Usually this is at about five weeks after infection but may be delayed months or years – some very few patients remaining seronegative for antibodies throughout the course of their HIV disease. As patients become ill with HIV disease the level of p24 antibody may fall and antigen may again become detectable in the serum.

Section 6: The HIV antibody test

The HIV antibody test is the main way that HIV is detected. As serological tests go it is highly reliable but it must always be remembered that screening tests, particularly the antiglobulin ELISA test, do generate some false positives and that any positive test result by any method should always be confirmed by a repeat test using a different method – preferably on a second sample in case tubes have been labelled in error. It must also be remembered that some patients do not raise an antibody response to HIV and thus a negative HIV antibody test is not an absolute reassurance that a patient is not infected.

Several different methods for detecting HIV antibodies are now available. The ELISA tests (Enzyme Linked Immuno Sorbent Assays) have the simplest methodology and are the easiest to perform (see 13, 14, 15) but the various viral antigens are not separated in these methods and thus separate estimation of antibodies to core and coat proteins is not possible.

The ELISA tests

There are at least three forms of ELISA test for HIV antibodies. The simplest, the antiglobulin assay (13), is performed in wells with HIV antigen fixed to the base of the well and prepared by lysing HIV infected malignant T-cells. The patient's serum is added to the wells and if antibodies are present they bind to the antigen. After washing, enzyme labelled antihuman immunoglobulin is added and followed after a further washing by the substrate for the enzyme label. A colour reaction occurs if HIV antibodies which were present in the patient's serum are bound in the well.

A second ELISA test is the competitive assay (14, 15), where again HIV antigen is fixed to the base of the well but both patient's serum and enzyme labelled anti-HIV antibodies are added to the well. If antibodies are present in the serum they bind to the antigen preventing the labelled anti-HIV antibodies from doing so and no colour reaction occurs. If antibodies are not present in the serum the enzyme labelled antibody binds to the antigen and a colour reaction appears but in this case indicates a negative test result (see 15).

The third form of ELISA, the capture assay (14), is when antihuman immunoglobulin coats the well and patient's serum is added. If anti-HIV antibodies are present in the serum they will adhere to the antihuman immunoglobulin and the addition of HIV antigen, and subsequently enzyme labelled anti-HIV antibody will result in a positive colour reaction.

The different ELISAs all have particular advantages but the competitive ELISA is the one used most frequently for screening for HIV antibodies in the United Kingdom as it has fewer false positive reactions than the antiglobulin assay. The capture assay is most commonly used as a confirmatory method and a minor change in its methodology allows anti-HIV IgM to be detected. In the United Kingdom the Western blot and RIPA methods tend to be used only for particularly difficult sera and in research laboratories.

13

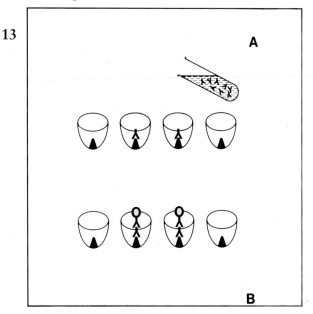

13 Schematic representation of the antiglobulin ELISA test. The dark triangles represent viral antigens and the Ys represent immunoglobulin molecules.

"ELISA" TESTS FOR HIV ANTIBODY

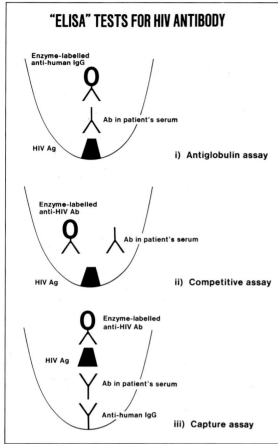

i) Antiglobulin assay

Enzyme-labelled anti-human IgG
Ab in patient's serum
HIV Ag

ii) Competitive assay

Enzyme-labelled anti-HIV Ab
Ab in patient's serum
HIV Ag

iii) Capture assay

Enzyme-labelled anti-HIV Ab
HIV Ag
Ab in patient's serum
Anti-human IgG

14 ELISA tests. This diagram compares the method of the antiglobulin ELISA test with the competitive and capture ELISA assays.

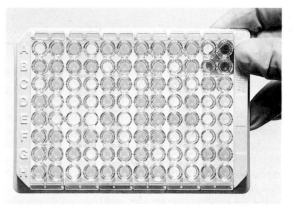

15 ELISA wells for a competitive ELISA assay. The clear wells indicating positive HIV antibody test result and the coloured wells indicating a negative result.

The immunofluorescent technique

In this method HIV infected lymphocytes are fixed to a microscope slide and patient's serum is applied. If anti-HIV antibodies are present in the serum they will adhere to the cells on the slide. After washing, fluorescent labelled antihuman immunoglobulin is applied to the slide and thus a positive result is seen to fluoresce. This method is simple but time consuming and requires more expertise than it does to work with ELISA kits. It also requires a fluorescent microscope. A similar method has also been employed using an enzyme label giving a coloured result visible to the naked eye on a slide (the Karpas test).

The agglutination assay

Recently yet another test method has been developed using latex beads coated with HIV antigen. When serum that contains HIV antibodies is added a positive reaction is indicated by agglutination of the latex beads. This test is technically simple and possibly will be cheap enough for application in the Third World (see **20**).

16 The HIV antibody agglutination assay. In this form of test latex beads coated with HIV antigen are added to the patient's serum. If HIV antibodies are present they result in agglutination of the latex beads.

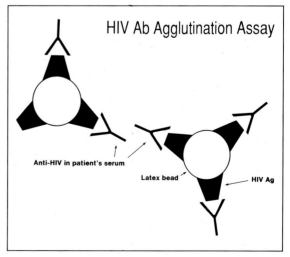

HIV Ab Agglutination Assay

Anti-HIV in patient's serum
Latex bead
HIV Ag

The Western blot and RIPA tests

These utilise gel electrophoresis to separate viral antigens and thus antibodies to individual proteins can be detected. This does not necessarily mean, however, that these tests are more sensitive than the ELISA tests.

17

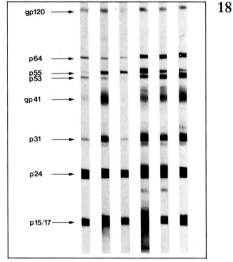

17 The Western blot method involves electrophoresis of disrupted HIV virions on slab gels. Most viral antigens can thus be individually detected. Cells in a malignant T cell line infected with HIV are lysed and the lysate is centrifuged and placed in wells on a polyacrylamide gel slab (A). Electrophoresis then separates the various proteins by molecular weight and charge. When this is complete the slab gel is placed adjacent to a nitrocellulose sheet and the viral proteins are 'blotted' upon it again using electrophoresis (B).

18

The patient's serum is then added to the nitrocellulose sheet and if HIV antibodies are present they will react with the viral antigens. After washing, labelled antihuman immunoglobulin is then applied and the 'Western blot' of the viral proteins is visualised.

18 Western blot results. Note that several viral proteins and glycoproteins are represented (see also 11).

19

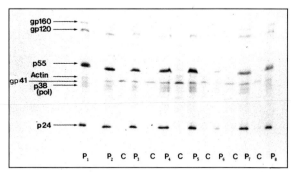

19 The RIPA Test (Radio Immune Precipitin Assay). This third form of HTLV III/LAV antibody testing is also highly reliable. The patient's serum is added to protein coated plastic beads and any immunoglobulin molecules present bind to the surface of the beads (A). Radioactive HTLV III/LAV infected malignant T-cell lysate (prepared by adding labelled methionine to cell culture) is added. Labelled HTLV III/LAV antigen binds to HTLV III/LAV antibody if present on the surface of the beads (B). Heat is then used to separate the antigen antibody

20

complexes are then seperated by electrophoresis in polyacrylamide gel (D). When this is complete, the gel with the separated radioactive viral antigens is placed against an x-ray plate and the RIPA result becomes visible (E).

20 Photograph of an x-ray plate of a RIPA result. Note that the line representing actin represents a cellular protein from the malignant T-cell line and not a viral component. It can be seen to be present in control sera as well as patients' sera.

Section 7: The origin of HIV

HIV seems likely to have originated in central Africa where serum samples from as early as the 1950s have been found to be seropositive. No serum samples stored in the United States prior to the 1970s have been found to be seropositive. Although HIV appears to have been present in Africa longer than in the United States, the rapidly rising incidence of cases in Africa also suggests a new epidemic.

Cases were occurring in Haiti before the USA, and this may have been due to the fact that migrant Haitian workers spent periods of time in central Africa in the 1960s and 1970s, and some returned to the homeland. In the 1970s Haiti was popular as a holiday resort for male homosexuals from the USA. Many early patients in Europe and Australasia appear to have contracted their infection in the USA. HIV is now epidemic worldwide.

In Africa the disease appears to have an equal incidence in both sexes, whereas in the western world the vast majority of cases have been homosexual men. This is because the virus was first introduced into this group and as homosexuals seldom have sex with women the disease has remained relatively restricted to this risk group.

There are, however, in the western world many documented cases of women contracting HIV infection from single episodes of vaginal intercourse with HIV infected men and there is little doubt that with time more and more cases will be seen in heterosexuals in the West. In areas where the virus has been spread by intravenous drug users, the majority of whom are heterosexual, spread to women and children has been more frequent. It appears that if a pregnant woman is HIV infected the chance of her infant being born with the infection is approximately 50%. Antenatal screening of HIV infected mothers will hopefully limit the incidence of paediatric AIDS.

Recently a second AIDS virus was discovered by Luc Montagnier's team in West Africa. Initially named LAV II it has been renamed HIV II. It appears to cause disease identical to HIV I, to spread in an identical fashion (and is likely to be equally sensitive to anti-viral drugs effective against HIV I). However, its genome varies some 30% from HIV I and a separate ELISA test using HIV II antigens is necessary to detect its presence when screening blood.

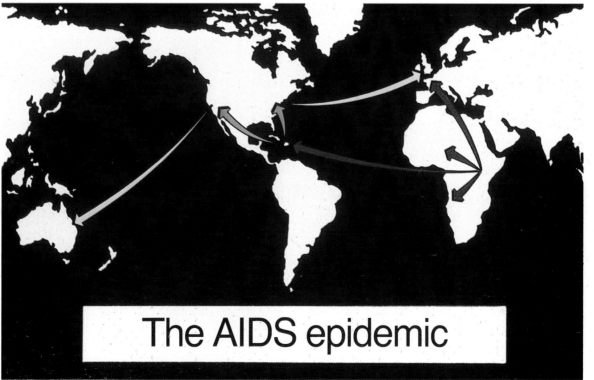

The AIDS epidemic

21 Map of the world showing probable origin and spread of HIV.

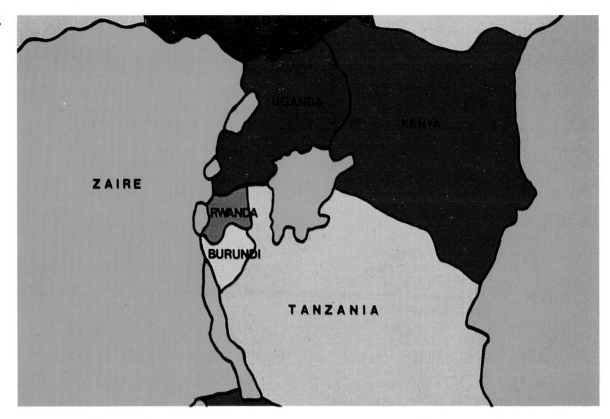

22 Map of central Africa showing countries of highest density of HIV disease. The highest incidence of AIDS in Africa appears to be in southern Uganda, and the small central African states of Ruanda and Burundi. In these countries the epidemic is known locally as 'slim disease'.

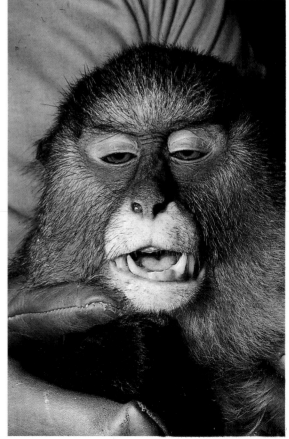

23

23 Wild caught African green monkeys have a very high incidence (60%) of infection with an immunodeficiency virus closely related to HIV called Simeon T Lymphotropic Virus type III (STLV III) or Simeon Immunodeficiency Virus (SIV). This virus does not appear to cause AIDS in the African green monkey, but when injected into Asian Macque monkeys from a different continent it results in AIDS. Probably the African green has, by a process of evolution (death of sensitive individuals and re-population with animals resistant to SIV), developed a natural resistance to the virus. In recent years the transfer of this or a related virus to the human population is the probable origin of the AIDS epidemic. How a transfer between species may have occurred is uncertain. The use of African green monkey blood in certain fertility rites is a possible explanation.

24

Immunodeficiency viruses

LAV	=	HTLV3	=	**HIV1**
LAV2	=	HTLV4	=	**HIV2**
		STLV3	=	**SIV**

24 Immunodeficiency viruses: LAV, HTLV III and HIV I are all names for the original AIDS virus. LAV II isolated from West Africa by the French has been renamed HIV II. LAV II is more closely related to the Simeon retrovirus (STLV III renamed SIV) than is HIV I. HTLV IV, isolated from humans in West Africa by a team from the USA, appears to be very closely related to SIV and is very similar to HIV II.

25

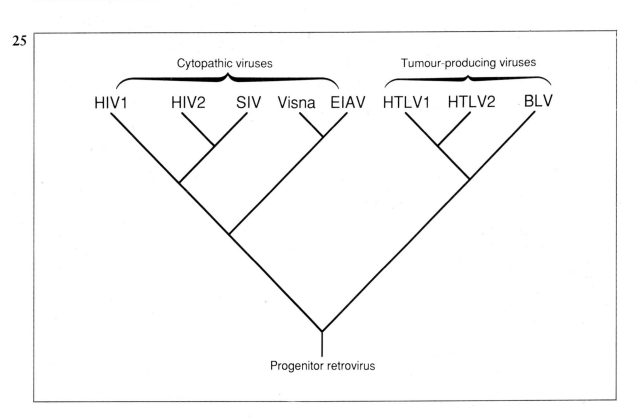

25 Retrovirus phylogeny. Proposed phylogeny of the retroviruses so far discovered. Interestingly, at some point in the revolution the retroviruses appear to have divided into two groups – those that cause cells to divide thus producing leukaemias and tumours such as HTLV I, the cause of human T-cell leukaemia; and those that cause cells to die off (cytopathic) such as HIV. The HIV genome is more closely related to the Visna virus (which causes degenerative brain disease in sheep and goats) than it is to the human virus HTLV I. HTLV II is not known to cause disease in man but has been isolated from a very few patients with hairy cell leukaemia.

EIAV = Equine Infectious Anaemia Virus
BLV = Bovine Leukaemia Virus

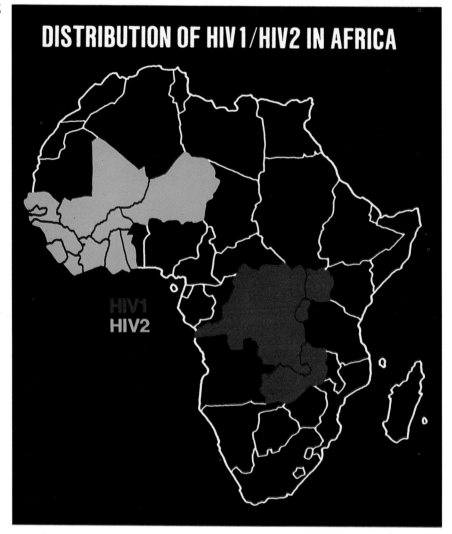

DISTRIBUTION OF HIV 1/HIV2 IN AFRICA

HIV1
HIV2

26 AIDS in Africa. Countries showing highest incidence of HIV I shaded in red, those where HIV II has first been isolated in green.

The true incidence of AIDS in Africa is very unclear as diagnostic facilities are less available and case reporting poor. The presentation of AIDS also differs with a gastrointestinal presentation being more common. To facilitate diagnosis in Africa a clinical case definition for AIDS in adults has been developed by the World Health Organisation. In Africa AIDS in an adult is defined by the existence of the two major signs of HIV infection and at least one minor sign in the absence of other known causes of immunosuppression such as cancer or severe malnutrition. The major signs are weight loss greater than 10% of body weight; chronic diarrhoea for longer than one month; and fever for longer than one month (intermittent or constant). The minor signs are persistent cough for longer than one month; general pruritic dermatitis; recurrent herpes zoster; oropharyngeal candidiasis; chronic progressive and disseminated herpes simplex infection; and generalised lymphadenopathy. The presence of disseminated Kaposi's sarcoma or cryptococcal meningitis are sufficient by themselves for the diagnosis of AIDS in Africa.

(Reference: Colebunders R et al. *Lancet* 1987; i: 492-493)

Section 8: The clinical spectrum and classification of HIV disease

It is now realised that so far the syndrome of AIDS has been seen in only a small proportion of those infected by HIV. Early in the epidemic perhaps only one in a hundred of those infected with HIV have actually developed the syndrome of AIDS. Other clinical syndromes have been defined:

Definitions

1. AIDS (see Section 4)
2. AIDS related complex (ARC)
3. Persistent generalised lymphadenopathy (PGL) (28)

27

Two clinical findings of HIV infection, plus two laboratory abnormalities suggestive of it.	
Clinical findings	**Laboratory abnormalities**
Fatigue	Decreased T-helper cell count
Night sweats	
	Increased serum globulins
Lymphadenopathy >3 months	
	Anergy
Weight loss (>10% total body weight)	Anaemia
Fever >3 months	
Diarrhoea	

28

Persistent generalised lymphadenopathy (PGL)

(i) Lymphadenopathy of at least three months duration involving two or more extra-inguinal sites.

(ii) Absence of any current illness or drug use known to cause lymphadenopathy.

(iii) Presence of reactive hyperplasia in a lymph if a biopsy is performed.

27 **The definition of the AIDS related complex,** unlike the definition of AIDS, is used loosely and means different things to different doctors. Most people, however, who are unwell from HIV disease with systemic symptoms but who have not had a major opportunistic infection or other AIDS diagnoses, will be found to fit the definition of ARC. Oral thrush, hairy leukoplakia and many other common problems in HIV disease are probably best included in the list of clinical findings. Also a positive HIV antigen test should probably be included in the list of laboratory abnormalities.

28 **PGL** was originally described as a syndrome in an effort to distinguish those people infected with the 'putative AIDS agent' from patients with lymphadenopathy from other causes. This rigid definition is less important now that HIV has been discovered and the HIV antibody test is available.

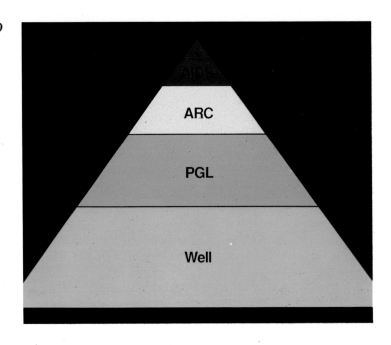

29 The total population of those infected with HIV.
A small proportion with AIDS, a larger proportion with ARC, but the majority only with lymphadeno-pathy or no sign of infection. AIDS represents only the tip of an iceberg in the 1980s – so early in the HIV epidemic.

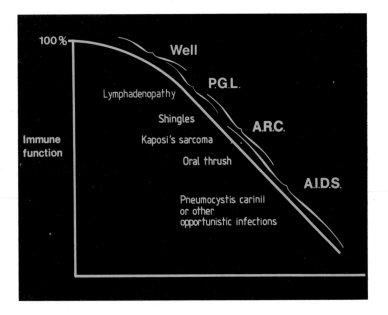

30 The decline in immune function with time. This graph shows the relationship of immune function to the various defined syndromes. Note the considerable overlap between the syndromes of ARC and AIDS. An ARC patient with oral thrush and weight loss may be considerably less well than an early AIDS patient with Kaposi's sarcoma and no oral thrush or weight loss.

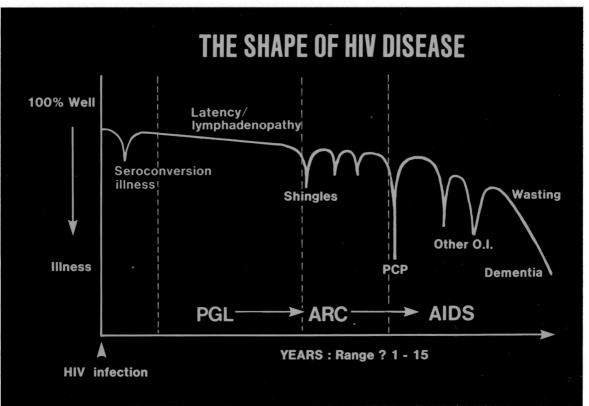

THE SHAPE OF HIV DISEASE

100% Well

Latency/
lymphadenopathy

Seroconversion
illness

Shingles

Wasting

Illness

Other O.I.

PCP

Dementia

PGL ⟶ ARC ⟶ AIDS

YEARS : Range ? 1 - 15

HIV infection

31   The shape of HIV disease. From this diagram it can be seen that for the first few years most patients with HIV infection remain well. Often the earliest ARC symptom is that of shingles. This may be followed by several minor infections before the first presentation of AIDS which is often with *Pneumocystis carinii* pneumonia (PCP) with which the patient may be severely ill but often makes a complete recovery. However, over the following year or two further episodes of severe infection of various kinds are likely to ensue, serious weight loss may set in and the final cause of death is often either a wasting syndrome or progressive HIV encephalopathy. This curve is drawn for a typical patient. However, the time from infection to death may be as short as a year or two or perhaps as long as ten or 20 years – the upper limit is not yet known. A patient may well die from his first episode of an opportunistic infection. The important point of the diagram is to try and illustrate that AIDS is more a state of risk rather than a single continuous illness. The patient suffers *episodes* of severe infection, being well for much of the intervening time. He is vulnerable to infection the whole time. The gradient of this curve is different from that of **30** which suggests a steady decline in immune function with time.

CDC Classification of HIV Disease

Group I

Acute Infection

Group II

Asymptomatic Infection

Group III

Progressive Generalised Lymphadenopathy

Group IV

Other Diseases :
a) Constitutional disease
b) Neurological disease
c) Secondary infectious diseases
   i. Specified secondary infectious diseases listed
      in the CDC Surveillance definition for AIDS.
   ii. Other specified secondary infectious disease.
d) Secondary cancers
e) Other conditions

32 **The CDC classification of HIV disease.** In an effort to classify HIV disease more sensibly than the crude syndromes of ARC and AIDS, the Center for Disease Control, Atlanta, Georgia, have produced the above classification system for HIV disease. This has been adopted by many hospitals but most physicians prefer to use the term ARC or AIDS simply to describe in detail what any particular patient is suffering from.

The Walter Reed staging classification for HIV infection

The Walter Reed staging system for HIV infection developed at the Walter Reed Army Institute in Washington DC stages HIV disease on immunological and clinical criteria. It is perhaps the most logical staging system for HIV disease – far better than the wide lumping of cases into "ARC" and "AIDS". Using this system of classification, after three years patients in all stages have moved on in classification by one or two stages. This might suggest that after a total of 18 years (3×6) the mortality of untreated HIV disease may approach 100%. To date, however, it is quite unknown what percentage of infected patients will develop AIDS. In groups that have been followed for five to six years some 30% have developed AIDS. Antiretroviral drugs that are now being introduced may also have an effect on disease progression.

Stage	HIV Ab or Ag or Isolation	Chronic Lymph-adenopathy	T-helper cells/mm^3	DTH	Thrush	O.I.
WR 0	−	−	> 400	Normal	−	−
WR 1	+	−	> 400	Normal	−	−
WR 2	+	+	> 400	Normal	−	−
WR 3	+	±	< 400	Normal	−	−
WR 4	+	±	< 400	Partial	−	−
WR 5	+	±	< 400	Anergy and/or +	−
WR 6	+	±	< 400	Anergy/Partial	±	+

33   The essential criteria for assignment to each stage are indicated by the squares. DTH denotes delayed type hypersensitivity and OI denotes opportunistic infection. Kaposi's sarcoma is not an important part of the staging system but is added as K, e.g. WR5K if present. B symptoms or constitutional symptoms (loss of greater than 10% of body weight, fevers, night sweats or chronic diarrhoea for longer than a month) are denoted by the addition of the letter B after the staging number. Other neoplasms are indicated by the addition of the letter N, and CNS symptoms by the addition of the letters CNS.

34

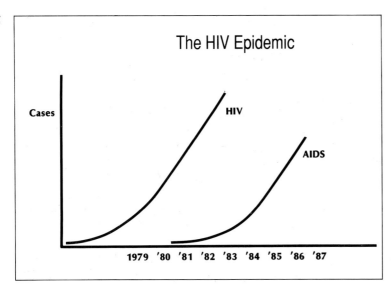

34 Survival curves in patients with Kaposi's sarcoma with and without opportunistic infections. A considerable proportion of patients with Kaposi's sarcoma without opportunistic infections survive for prolonged periods. This probably indicates that Kaposi's sarcoma, in most patients who get it, occurs relatively earlier in the course of HIV disease than the majority of opportunistic infections.

35

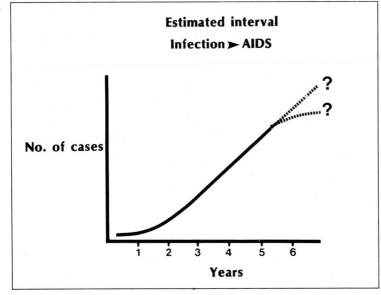

35 Lagtime infection → AIDS. These double curves indicate that the spread of HIV through a community precedes the spread of AIDS by several years due to the long incubation period. This has serious social implications in that HIV may spread widely within a community before disease is apparent and precautions are taken.

36

Estimated interval

Infection ➤ AIDS

No. of cases

| 1 | 2 | 3 | 4 | 5 | 6 |

Years

36 Incubation period. The interval between infection with HIV to development of AIDS is very variable. The incubation period may vary from eight months to six years or more. Over the last six years that the epidemic has been followed, a constant proportion of infected individuals has developed AIDS each year. It is uncertain whether this trend will continue or whether this proportion will tail off to give an average incubation of perhaps four to six years.

Part 2 Clinical manifestations of HIV disease

Introduction

HIV disease may first present with a seroconversion illness within a few weeks of infection with the virus. Seroconversion is asymptomatic in the majority of individuals and the first clinical manifestations of HIV disease may not develop for some years (see 31). Usually constitutional symptoms such as fatigue and night sweats and relatively minor medical problems such as shingles and oral thrush precede the development of major opportunistic infections or tumours. At this stage the patient does not satisfy the CDC criteria for AIDS (see Appendix A) but is said to be suffering from the AIDS related complex (for ARC definition see Section 8).

The full blown syndrome of AIDS may not develop for some months or years in the patient with ARC and most commonly presents with an interstitial pneumonia (*Pneumocystis carinii* pneumonia accounts for some 65% of first presentations of AIDS), Kaposi's sarcoma, primary or secondary central nervous system disease, dysphagia, diarrhoea, lymphoma or pyrexia from a disseminated opportunistic infection such as *Mycobacterium avium intracellulare* (MAI).

AIDS however may present *de novo* in a previously clinically well HIV antibody positive patient. This is more often true when the presenting illness of AIDS is Kaposi's sarcoma. However, *Pneumocystis* pneumonia may occasionally present suddenly in very fit looking individuals.

The 'minor' manifestations of HIV disease such as fatigue, lymphadenopathy, night sweats, weight loss, chronic diarrhoea, oral cavity disease, skin disease, ENT problems and thrombocytopenia, although seldom life threatening or requiring hospital admission, are very important in both diagnosis and management. Recognition of these problems, which may be very subtle, allows early diagnosis of HIV disease and their treatment may provide the patient with considerable symptomatic relief.

These minor problems are also important in assessing disease progression. A previously well HIV antibody positive individual who develops constitutional symptoms, first one and then perhaps others, is obviously progressing in his HIV disease. Recognition of this may result in the physician instituting some antiretroviral treatment at a time when it may be hoped to result in greatest benefit for the patient.

In this part we discuss the clinical manifestations of HIV disease under twelve different sections, mostly dealing with different organ systems of the body. We have not divided this clinical section into separate sections for ARC and AIDS as these are arbitrary divisions imposed on a single disease process. For example, people with HIV disease are more susceptible to many different infectious diarrhoeas. Some of the diarrhoeal infections satisfy CDC criteria for AIDS – others do not. We have dealt with them all under the heading of gastrointestinal disease. Diseases that satisfy CDC criteria for AIDS are generally referred to in the text as doing so. If there is doubt, however, reference to Appendix A will establish whether a certain illness defines a patient as having AIDS or not.

Section 9: HIV seroconversion illness or 'acute HIV disease'

The patient presents acutely unwell with fever, rash, sore throat, tender lymphadenopathy and headache. This may be accompanied by clinical signs of meningitis or encephalitis. If a lumbar puncture is performed a raised CSF lymphocyte count suggestive of aseptic meningitis may be found. Usually the patient spontaneously recovers within a week. It is not known what percentage of patients who become infected with HIV develop this seroconversion illness or 'acute HIV disease'. We see it rarely however and thus think, for the most part, that this illness is asymptomatic or relatively minor, the patient assuming that he perhaps has a cold or influenza and not taking himself to the doctor.

37

38

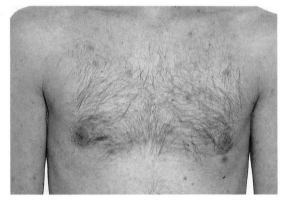
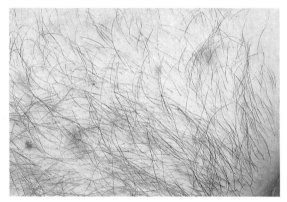

37 and 38   HIV seroconversion rash in a 22-year-old man who seroconverted five weeks after presentation with fever, sore throat, headache and the appearance of this eruption.

39

40

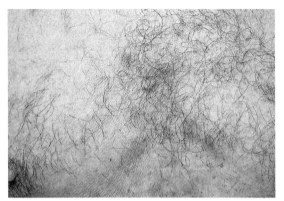

39 and 40   HIV seroconversion rash in a 45-year-old man. HIV serology was negative at the time this eruption was observed when the patient was acutely unwell with fever and headache. Seroconversion was noted six weeks later.

41

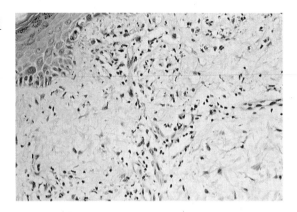

41   Skin biopsy in the patient shown above (**39, 40**). Histopathology shows a pattern of venulitis with extravasation of red cells and nuclear dusting.

Section 10: Lymphadenopathy

Generalized lymphadenopathy that has persisted for more than three months in a homosexual patient is very likely to be due to HIV disease. It is so common a finding that lymph node biopsy is no longer a routine practice if the patient is HIV antibody positive.

Biopsy is recommended to exclude lymphoma or tuberculous adenitis if the patient has prominent constitutional symptoms such as malaise and night sweats, is seronegative or has nodes which feel atypical. Usually lymphadenopathy in HIV disease feels rubbery and the nodes are mobile. If nodes are hard or fixed or are enlarging rapidly in one particular area they should be biopsied.

Usually lymphadenopathy secondary to HIV disease is non-tender but quite frequently patients will present with an increase in size of their lymph nodes which have become tender and they complain of fatigue at the same time. Patients often report that this occurs at times of heavy stress and work in their lives.

This 'glandular fever' syndrome is common and may be recurrent. The cause is unknown but is possibly due to minor flare-ups of systemic cytomegalovirus (CMV) infection. Usually the increased nodal swelling and fatigue subsides with rest.

The lymphadenopathy of HIV disease often regresses with time and progression of the disease.

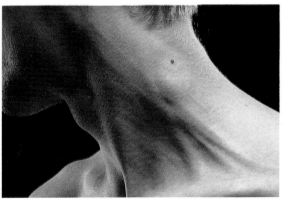

42   **Visible lymph node** in the neck of a patient with persistent generalized lymphadenopathy. Interestingly this patient had HIV seronegative PGL for three years, before seroconversion. He remains well after eight years of PGL, except for the recent development of seborrhoeic dermatitis.

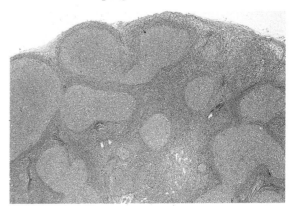

43   **Section of lymph node** showing extensive follicular hyperplasia. This is the typical finding in PGL but is a nonspecific finding seen in many reactive viral lymphadenopathies (H & E ×10).

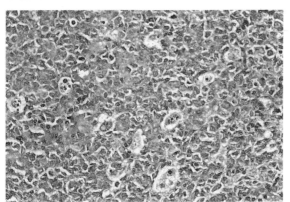

44   **Reactive centre of node** shown in **123** (higher power). Note the irregularly nucleated small and large lymphoid cells (centrocytes) and blast cells (H & E ×100).

45   **Section of lymph node** showing follicular depletion (H & E ×10). Follicular depletion is considered a poor prognostic sign and is often seen in the nodes of patients with AIDS. When seen in patients with PGL rapid progression to AIDS frequently occurs.

Section 11: Weight loss

Progressive weight loss is a manifestation of late HIV disease (whether it is occurring in a patient with ARC or AIDS) and may be extremely marked in some patients. The cause is uncertain but may in part be related to malabsorption. It is a very poor prognostic sign. Since September 1st 1987 a chronic wasting syndrome (greater than or equal to 10% weight loss plus either diarrhoea or fever for one month) in the presence of HIV seropositivity satisfies the CDC criteria for AIDS.

46

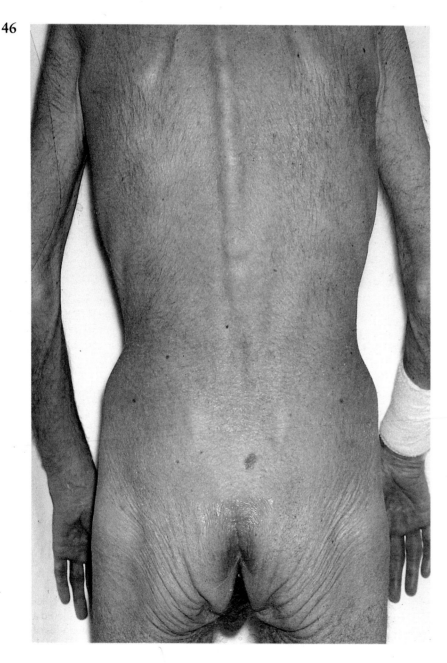

46 **Severe wasting** in a patient with AIDS.

Section 12: Oral cavity disease

Introduction

Oral cavity problems are extremely common in later stage HIV disease (ARC and AIDS).

Oral thrush and hairy leukoplakia are important clinical clues to the diagnosis of HIV and indicate that the disease has advanced to the stage where the development of AIDS, if it has not already occurred, is almost certain to do so within two years. 60-80% of patients with HIV disease presenting with oral thrush or hairy leukoplakia develop AIDS within two years.

Both thrush and leukoplakia are fairly specific signs of HIV disease: oral thrush is extremely uncommon in young people with their own teeth who are not diabetic and hairy leukoplakia has not been described outside of HIV disease.

Kaposi's sarcoma frequently first presents on the hard palate and this is dealt with in Section 15. Gingivitis is an extremely common problem in HIV disease and may lead to marked erosion of the gingiva. Although a major management problem in HIV disease, it is less useful diagnostically as gingivitis is common in the general population.

Aphthous ulceration is less common but may produce considerable morbidity with large painful ulcers on the soft palate and can persist for many months. Dental abscesses and intraoral warts seem to occur more commonly in patients with HIV infection than in the general population.

Table: *Oral cavity problems in HIV disease*

Oral thrush
Hairy leukoplakia
Kaposi's sarcoma
Gingivitis
Aphthous ulceration
Dental abscesses
Intraoral warts

Oral thrush in HIV disease

Oral thrush usually appears as white plaques on the hard and soft palate and the buccal surfaces. Sometimes the underlying mucosa is of normal colour (47), other times an angry red (48). If it is red the mouth may be uncomfortable. Occasionally the appearance is just of a beefy red oral mucosa with no white plaques, when it may be referred to as 'erythematous candidiasis'. In minor involvement white plaques are often seen first behind the second molar teeth (49). Oral thrush is easy to treat using either topical oral preparations that are not absorbed (such as mystatin pastilles, amphotericin B lozenges or miconazole gel) or systemic preparations (such as ketoconazole tablets). In cases of heavy infection with oral thrush, and in cases of oesophageal candidiasis, systemic treatments will usually be required. The hepatic toxicity of ketoconazole is extremely rare but liver function tests should be monitored. Many patients with ARC and AIDS require ketoconazole continuously to prevent recurrence of uncomfortable oral or oesophageal candidiasis.

47

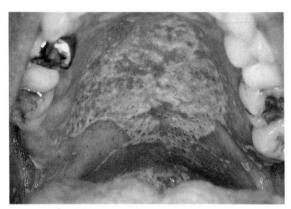

47 **Oral thrush** in a patient with AIDS with normal underlying oral mucosa.

48

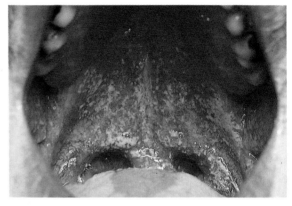

48 **Oral thrush** in a patient with AIDS with inflamed underlying oral mucosa.

49

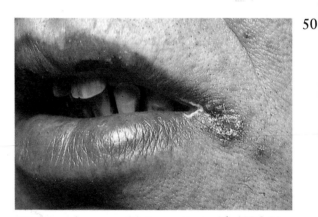

49 **Early oral thrush** in a patient with ARC.

50

50 **Angular stomatitis** in a patient with AIDS. Very frequently this painful cracking at the corners of the mouth is associated with oral thrush. It responds well to regular application of hydrocortisone 1% cream in combination with an antifungal such as miconazole. The oral thrush should also be treated.

Hairy leukoplakia in patients with HIV disease

These four pictures show different examples of hairy leukoplakia. The appearance is that of a ribbed whiteness along the sides of the tongue. It is usually asymptomatic although sometimes patients will complain of its appearance. Very occasionally it is painful. The term 'hairy' derives from the histopathological appearance of hairy projections of keratinised squamous epithelium. The white appearance is due to the keratinisation of the squamous epithelium leading to a soggy white skin on the surface of the tongue. The cause appears to be due to a proliferation of Epstein-Barr virus in the superficial layers of the squamous epithelium of the tongue (**55** to **58**).

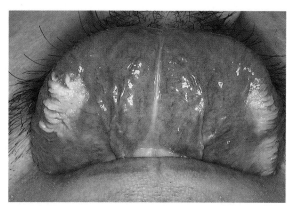

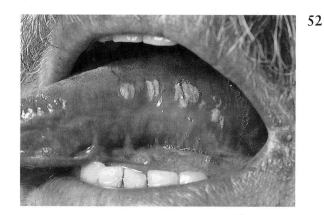

51 to 54   Hairy leukoplakia in patients with ARC and AIDS. Note the distinctive ribbed appearance.

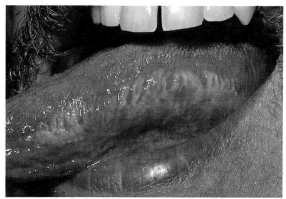
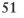

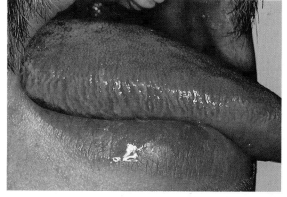

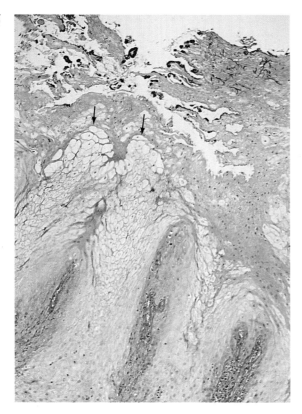

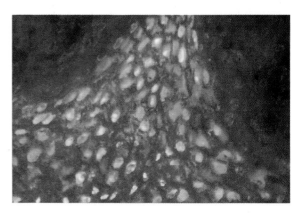

56 Immunofluorescent preparation using polyclonal antibody against Epstein-Barr virus (EBV) showing positive immunofluorescence in vacuolated cells in upper epithelium.

55 **Section of tongue with hairy leukoplakia,** showing vacuolated cells (arrows) suggesting viral infection. (H & E ×25)

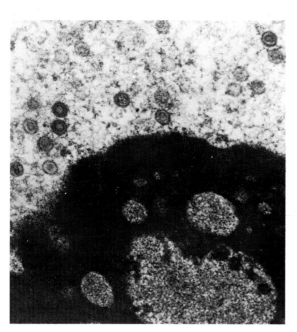

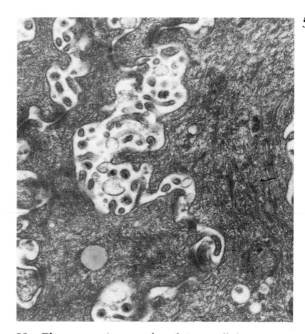

57 Electron micrograph of nucleus of infected squamous epithelial cell, showing condensed chromatin surrounded by multiple EBV particles. (×67,000)

58 Electron micrograph of intercellular spaces showing multiple EBU particles, some budding from the cell walls (×28,000). (Same patient as **57**.)

Gingivitis in patients with HIV disease

Recurrent painful bleeding gums with erosion of the gingiva is common in HIV disease. Regular dental hygiene with removal of plaque is essential. Betidine mouthwash may be used as a treatment or prophylaxis. Flare-ups usually respond to penicillin and metronidazole.

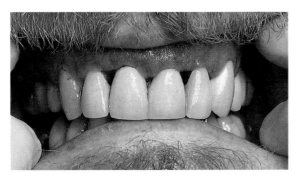
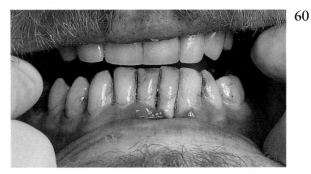

59 and 60 **Gingival erosion** in a young patient with AIDS.

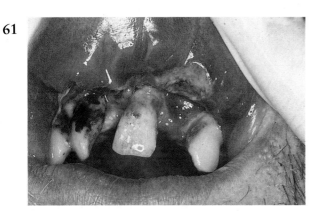
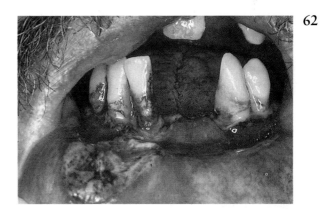

61 and 62 **Acute erosive gingivitis** in a patient with ARC.

Aphthous ulceration in HIV disease

Aphthous ulcers most commonly occur on the soft palate and are particularly painful. Topical application of triamcinolone acetonide 0.1% in orabase may help but this is difficult to apply to the soft palate. Very resistant cases, which may result in the patient's inability to eat, usually respond to thalidomide (see Appendix B).

63
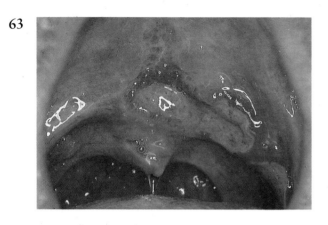

64
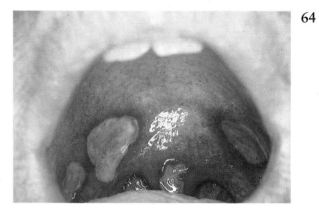

65
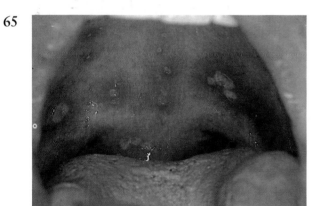

66
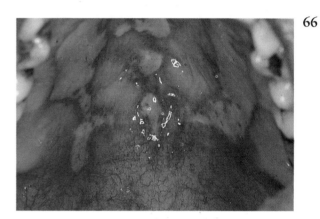

63 to 66   Aphthous ulceration in patients with AIDS.

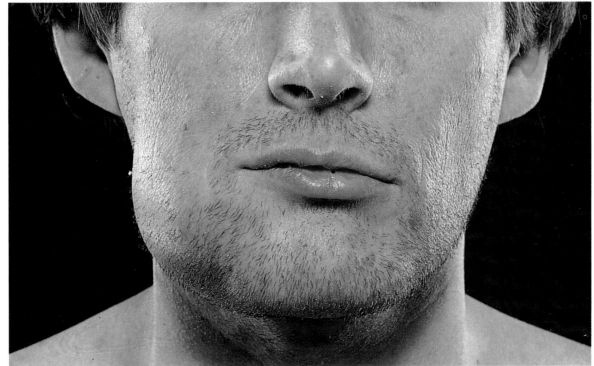

67   Dental abscess in a patient with ARC.

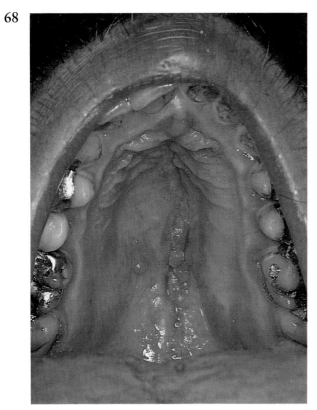

68 Intraoral warts in a patient with ARC.

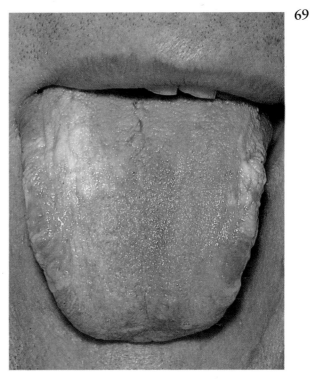

69   Coated tongue in a patient with ARC – a common nonspecific finding.

Section 13: Skin disease

Introduction

Often the first clinical manifestation of HIV disease is a skin eruption. The following skin eruptions are commonly seen:

1. Seborrhoeic dermatitis
2. Papulopruritic eruptions/folliculitis
3. Xeroderma (dry skin)
4. Shingles ⎫
5. Herpes simplex ⎬ viral skin eruptions
6. Molluscum contagiosum ⎭
7. Tineas (fungal skin and nail eruptions)

Seborrhoeic dermatitis

Seborrhoeic dermatitis, papulopruritic eruption and xeroderma are of uncertain origin although it is thought that overgrowth or sensitivity to the *Pityrosporum* yeasts may play an important part in the aetiology of the seborrhoeic dermatitis. Histopathology of the papulopruritic eruption suggests a vasculitic origin and the xeroderma may be in part caused by malabsorption of fatty acids. Depressed cellular immunity explains the viral and fungal skin eruptions.

There are many other skin eruptions that have been reported as occurring more frequently in HIV disease such as drug hypersensitivity rashes, impetigo and psoriasis. Other less frequently seen skin problems are reviewed at the end of this section.

Seborrhoeic dermatitis is most frequently seen on the face. Although a common eruption in the general population it is frequently more severe in HIV disease and often has never been a problem before in an HIV positive patient. The classical eruption on the face (**70** and **71**) involves the nasolabial folds and should certainly serve as a clinical pointer to AIDS in a patient presenting with chest infection, diarrhoea or central nervous system disease. When less severe it may only involve the eyebrow (**72**) or moustache area (**73**).

This rash responds well to hydrocortisone 1% cream in combination with an antifungal such as miconazole. Occasionally patients may be sensitive to such creams and ketoconazole cream is another alternative. A rash on the face is often very disturbing for a patient.

Seborrhoeic dermatitis may well spread more extensively on the body when it probably heralds a poor prognosis. The most frequent sites to be involved are the upper outer arms and the central chest area. On close inspection of the eruption it can be seen that many areas are not confluent but show follicular accentuation.

70
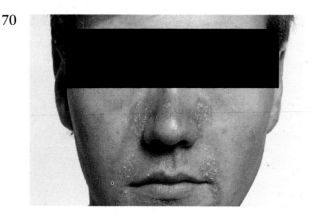

71
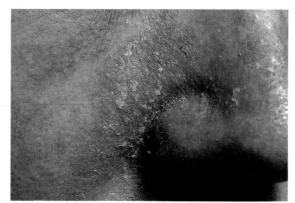

70 and **71** Florid seborrhoeic dermatitis on the face of a patient with ARC.

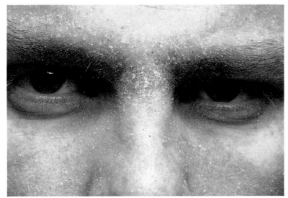

72

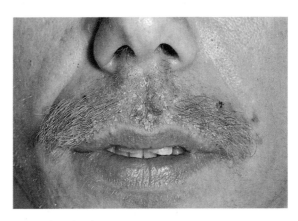

73

72 Seborrhoeic dermatitis involving the eyebrows in a patient with ARC.

73 Seborrhoeic dermatitis involving the moustache area in a patient with AIDS.

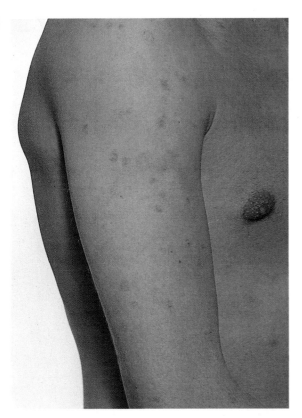

74

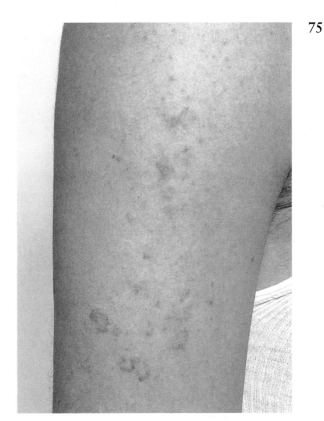

75

74 and 75 Numular seborrhoides on the upper arms. A pattern of seborrhoeic dermatitis frequently seen in HIV disease.

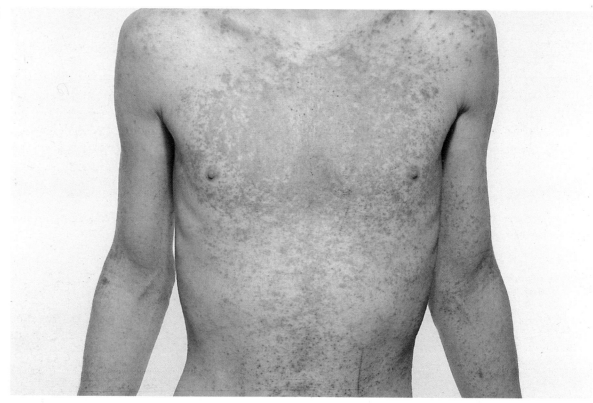

76 Seborrhoeic dermatitis of the chest spreading beyond the usual central sternal area.

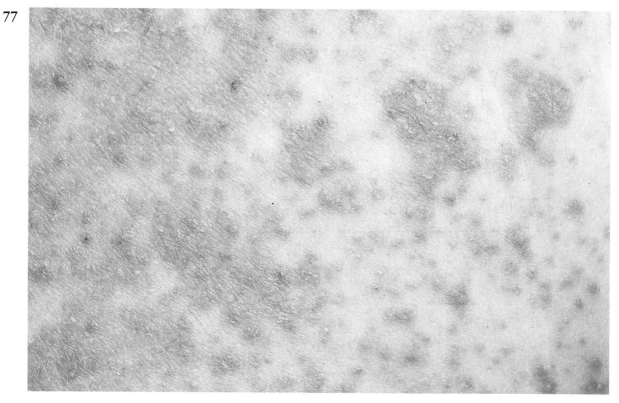

77 Close-up of the patient in **76** showing follicular accentuation.

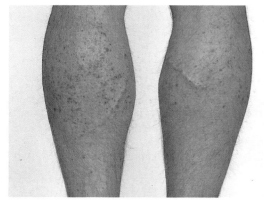

78 Extensive follicular dermatitis.

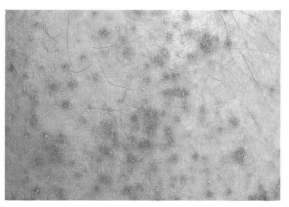

79 Close-up of 78.

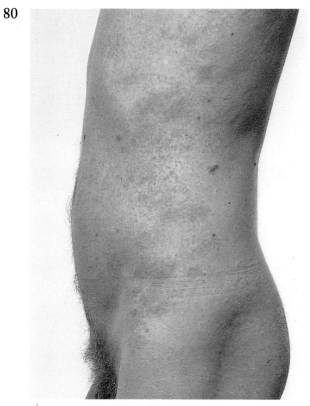

80 Extensive follicular dermatitis in a patient with AIDS (note the small Kaposi lesion on the flank).

81 Close-up of the patient in 80.

Papulopruritic eruption (folliculitis)

A papulopruritic eruption or 'itchy folliculitis' is the most frequent and most irritating of the skin eruptions in HIV disease. The lesions are small and clinically unimpressive without marked surrounding erythema. They are usually intensely pruritic and very frequently excoriated. The commonest sites are chest, upper arms, lateral neck and face, scalp, axillae and thighs. A few lesions that the clinician is likely to dismiss may cause a patient considerable distress.

Follicular lesions are usually culture negative. Histopathology may reveal a pattern of vasculitis.

Unfortunately the condition is very resistant to treatment but strong topical corticosteroids and antihistamines may provide some relief. For most patients the condition is an intermittent one. In Africa it is said that this eruption accounts for 30% of presentations of HIV disease and this may be because black skin is somewhat more pruritic than white skin.

82
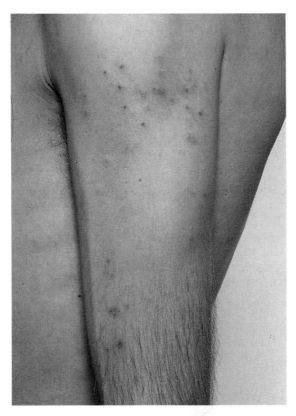

83
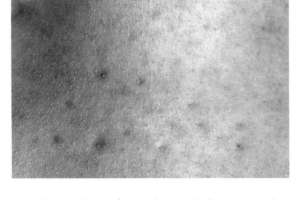

82 and **83** **Typical papulopruritic lesions** on the upper outer arm and central chest of the same patient. Note the excoriated lesions particularly on the arm. The 'seborrhoeic' areas are the commonest sites for this eruption.

84

84   Close-up of the eruption in **84** showing definite follicular lesions.

85
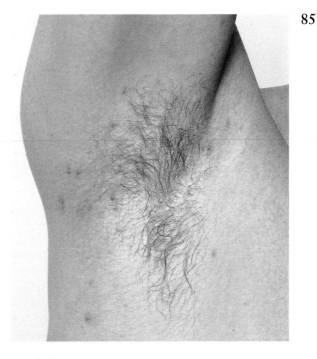

85   **Folliculitis** in the axillae is sometimes seen.

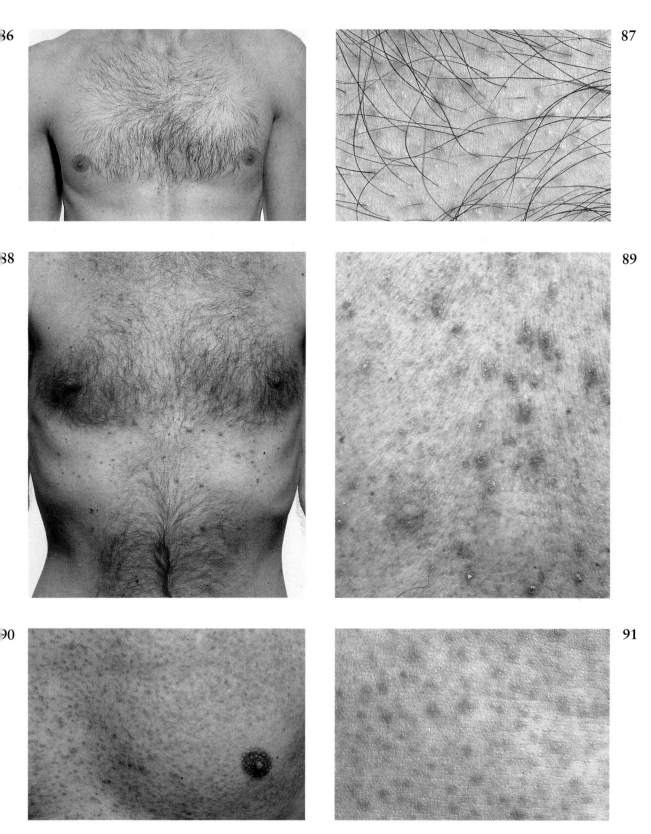

86 to **91** **Papulopruritic eruption** on the chest of three different patients with close-ups showing the varied morphology.

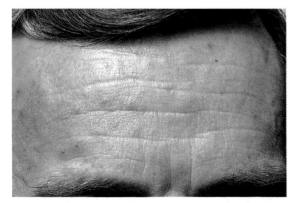

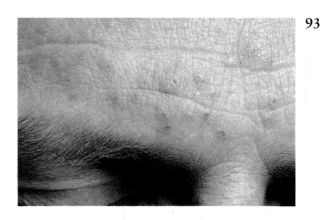

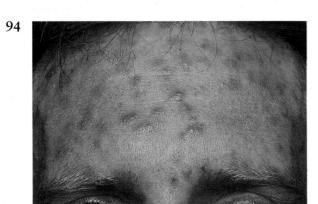

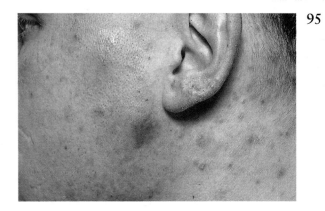

92 to 95 **A papulopruritic eruption** on the face is often excoriated, may be very prominent as in **94**, and is often noted behind the ear, as in **95**.

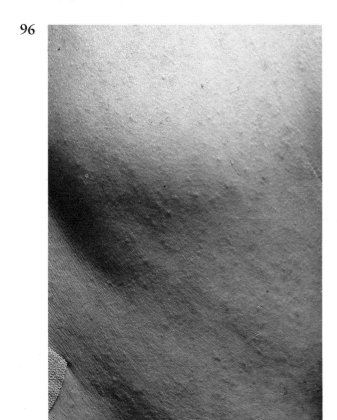

96 and 97 **A papulopruritic eruption** may be very subtle to the eye. This patient with these very small lesions had an intense pruritus.

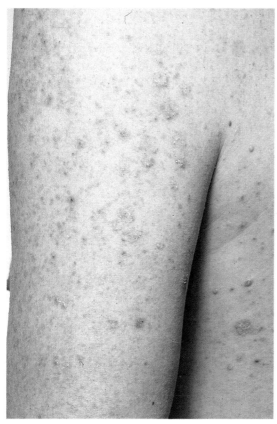

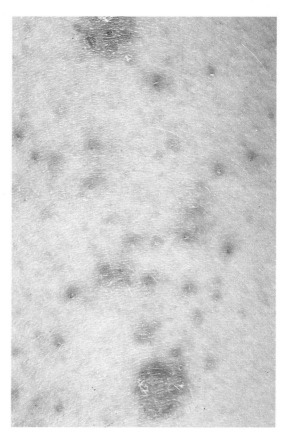

98 to 100 These pictures show a mixture of follicular and eczematous lesions occurring together. 99 is a close-up of the patient in 98.

This discoid eczema in 100 occurred in a patient who had had intense pruritus with only small lesions previously (see 92) before this more florid eruption appeared.

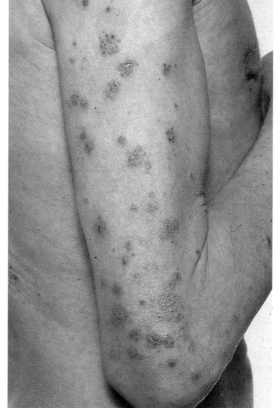

Xeroderma (dry skin)

Dry skin is almost universal in late stage HIV disease. It may be associated with pruritus. The cause is uncertain but may be related to malabsorption of fatty acids leading to apparent premature aging of the skin.

Considerable symptomatic relief can be provided by the regular use of bath oils, emollient soaps and copious quantities of moisturising creams.

101

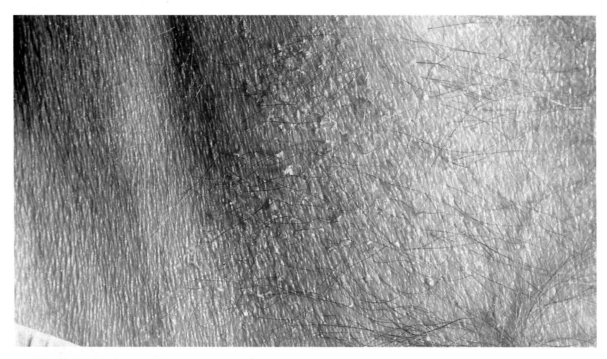

101 Dry skin on the flank of an AIDS patient.

102

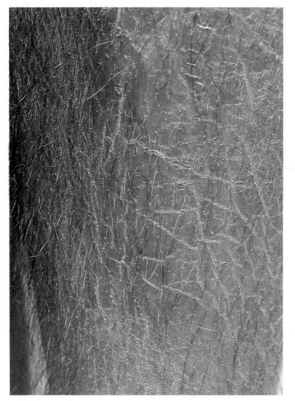

102 Dry skin on the shin of a 22-year-old patient with ARC. The appearance is one of 'asteatotic eczema' such as might be seen in the pretibial region of a man in his 70s or 80s.

Shingles

Shingles is often the first manifestation of immuno-suppression in patients with HIV disease. Shingles in a young at-risk individual should raise the strong suspicion of HIV disease but it should be remembered that shingles can sometimes occur spontaneously in normal healthy young people. In HIV disease shingles should be treated with high dose acyclovir treatment (800 mg five times a day for a week) because there is a significant incidence of zoster meningitis if left untreated. Treated or untreated the shingles usually resolves in a normal sequence and is not especially severe.

Dissemination is unusual but the shingles may occur in more than one dermatome at the same time (**105**). Interestingly, when chicken pox occurs in HIV positive patients the course is usually benign and not severe as one might expect in an immunocompromised adult. However, disseminated zoster without shingles has rarely been seen in severely ill AIDS patients (134-136).

03

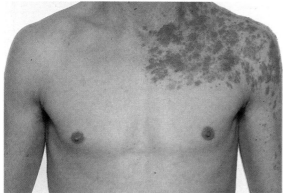

05

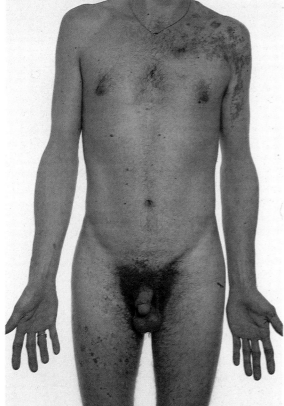

104

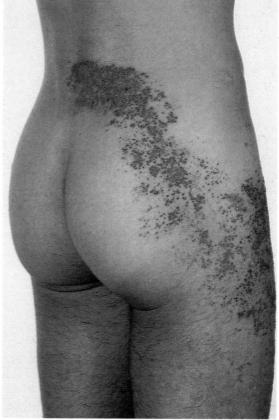

103   **Shingles** in the C4 dermatome in a patient with ARC.

104   **Shingles** in the L3 dermatome in a patient with AIDS.

105   **Shingles** in two dermatomes simultaneously (C4 and L2) in a patient with ARC. Two years after this presentation the patient died of cryptococcal meningitis.

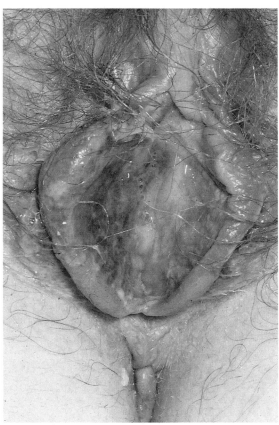

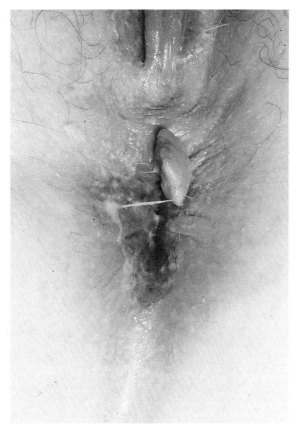

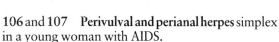

106 and 107 **Perivulval and perianal herpes** simplex in a young woman with AIDS.

Herpes simplex

Herpes simplex poses a considerable problem in HIV disease. Like HIV, HSV is a sexually transmitted virus and thus the majority of HIV infected patients are also herpes sufferers. As the immunosuppression of HIV disease increases patients are likely to have more severe and more frequent herpes attacks. Some may develop clinical herpes for the first time even though they may have been carrying the virus for many years.

The most frequent site in homosexual men is perianal herpes where the diagnosis may be difficult as lesions may be small and atypical and merely resemble a small perianal tear. The diagnostic clue is the severe pain. Herpes proctitis may accompany the skin lesions or may occur in isolation – it is also usually very painful. Treatment is acyclovir (200 mg five times a day for five to seven days) and probably should be instituted whenever an HIV antibody positive homosexual man complains of perianal pain. Some patients require continuous acyclovir (200 mg twice a day up to continuous full dose therapy) to remain lesion-free. In some patients with AIDS, however, herpes may continue to be a very benign disease despite the immunosuppression. Continuous muco-cutaneous ulceration from herpes simplex for more than a month satisfies the CDC criteria for AIDS – see Appendix A.

Perianal warts

Papillomavirus is also commonly a sexually transmitted disease and particularly in homosexual males perianal warts are common. HIV disease appears to make patients more susceptible to warts but not greatly so. Always difficult to treat, perianal warts in HIV positive patients are even more likely to recur after treatment.

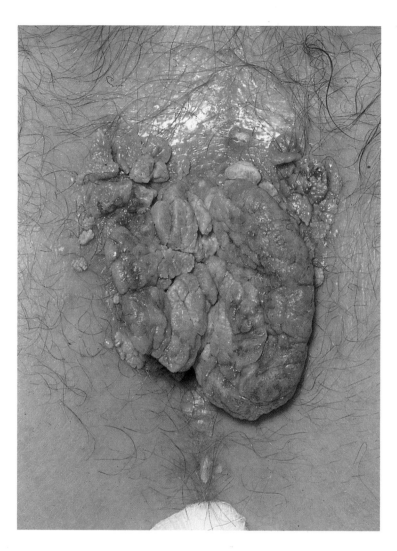

108 Perianal warts: A particularly severe case in a patient with HIV disease.

Molluscum contagiosum

Patients with HIV disease are particularly susceptible to molluscum contagiosum lesions – more so than they are to warts. Molluscum lesions may spread across the face possibly assisted by shaving. This produces a distinctive appearance rarely seen in any other disease and could be considered diagnostic of HIV disease. Widespread molluscum contagiosum implies a severely immunocompromised patient and a poor prognosis.

The lesions are difficult to treat. Classical treatment is to prick the lesions with a sharpened orange stick dipped in phenol. This is particularly painful on the face and an alternative, which leads to less recurrence, is to curette and cauterise lesions under local anaesthesia or to touch the lesions with cautery without anaesthesia. The lesions may respond to freezing with liquid nitrogen.

109
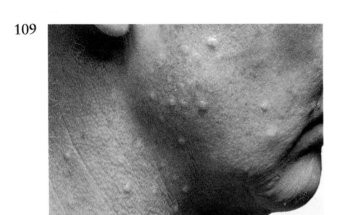

110
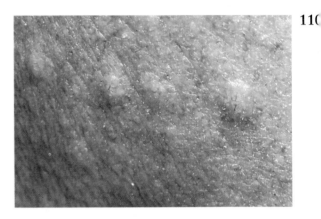

111
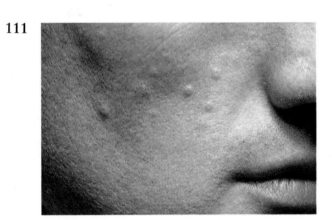

112
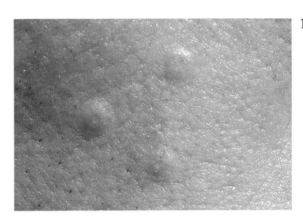

113
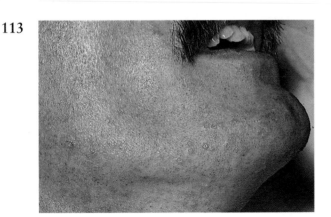

109 to 113 Molluscum contagiosum lesions on the face of AIDS patients. **110** is a close-up of the patient in **109**, and **112** a close-up of the patient in **111**.

Dermatophyte infections

Tinea pedis, tinea corporis and tinea unguum are all very common in patients with HIV disease and respond to conventional therapies. An inflammatory response to the fungus is often quite pronounced (115) despite the immunocompromise. However, tinea incognito may occur (117). Topical antifungals work well. For tinea unguum systemic antifungals are required, e.g. ketoconazole 200 mg b.d. (griseofulvin is an alternative but HIV disease patients frequently show allergy to this drug). Candidal intertrigo is also seen in HIV disease (120) and HIV should probably be considered as well as diabetes when candidal intertrigo is seen in the general population.

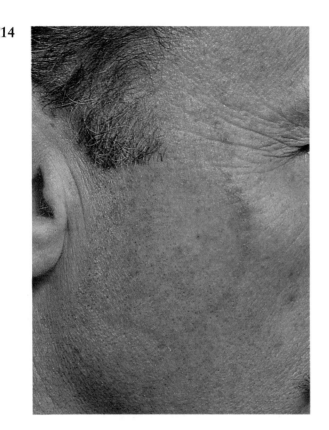

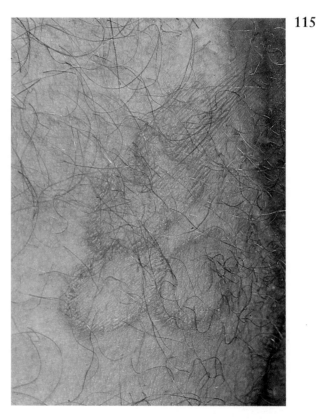

114 **Dermatophyte infection** on the face of a patient with ARC.

115 **Tineas rubrum** infection on the thigh of a young man with ARC.

116

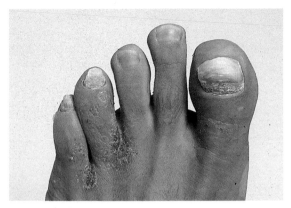

116 **Aggressive tinea pedis and tinea unguum** on the foot of an AIDS patient.

118

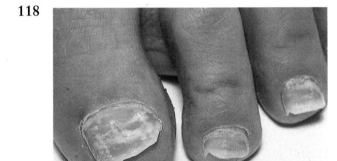

117

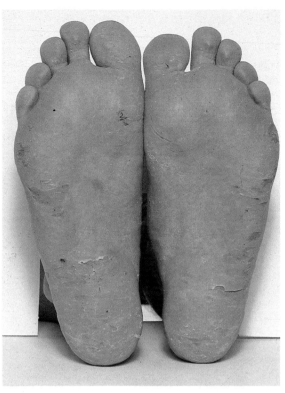

117 **Extensive dermatophyte involvement** of the soles of both feet in a patient with AIDS (skin scrapings positive for fungus).

119

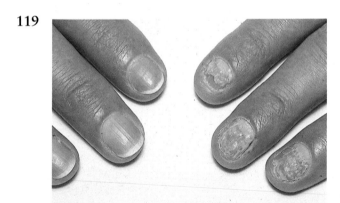

118 and 119 **Tinea unguum** involving toenails and fingernails in a patient with ARC.

120

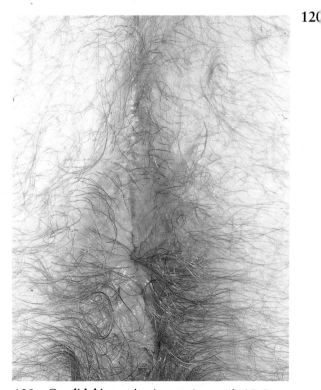

120 **Candidal intertrigo** in a patient with ARC.

Other less common skin eruptions in HIV disease

Patients with HIV disease seem to be more susceptible to streptococcal infections including streptococcal sore throat, *Strep. pneumoniae* infections, streptococcal adenitis, impetigo and cellulitis.

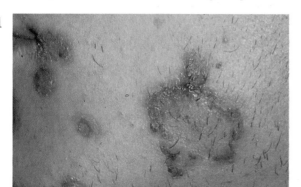

121 **Impetigo** in an ARC patient spreading from an area of angular cheilitis.

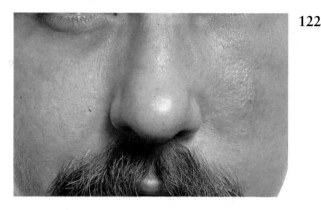

122 **Cellulitis (erysipelas)** on the face of a patient with ARC. This failed to respond to oral therapy and intravenous antibiotics were required.

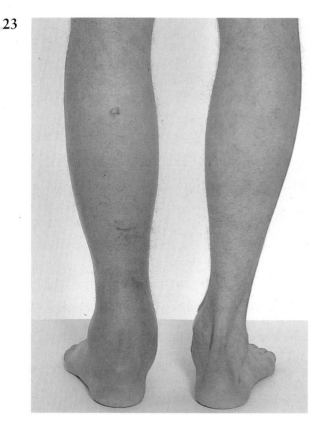

123 **The cellulitis** on this patient's left lower leg (note erythema and oedema) was the presenting problem of his HIV disease. When examined for the cellulitis small Kaposi lesions were noted on the leg.

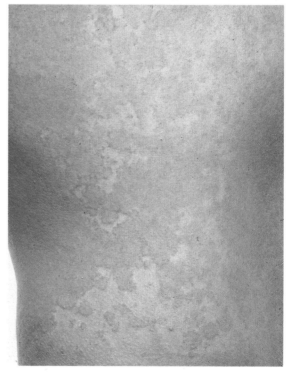

124 **Drug eruption** in a patient with AIDS being treated with cotrimoxazole for PCP. Sensitivity to various drugs (especially cotrimoxazole and griseofulvin) seems to be much more frequent in HIV disease. This is often associated with a febrile reaction. In cases that are not too severe therapy with cotrimoxazole, for example, can be continued with the concurrent use of an antihistamine such as terfenadine.

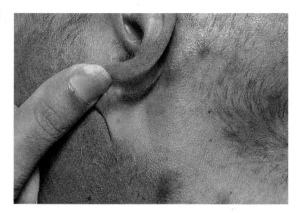

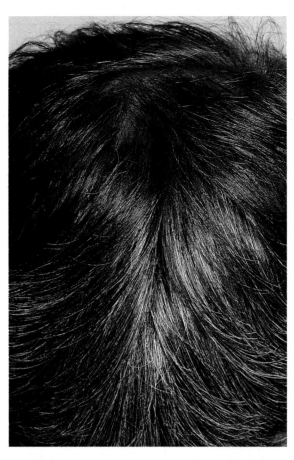

125 Pigmentation. This patient developed phototoxic hyperpigmentation following VP16 systemic chemotherapy for Kaposi's sarcoma. Hyperpigmentation in the sun-exposed areas is often seen in late stage HIV disease and is most probably due to drug therapies such as long-term ketoconazole treatment but could be a manifestation of the disease itself or one of the opportunistic infections (possibly MAI).

126 Premature greying of the hair is frequently seen in HIV disease.

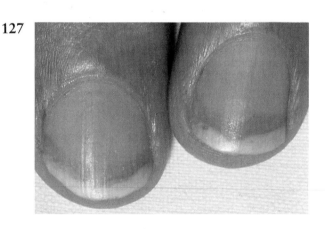

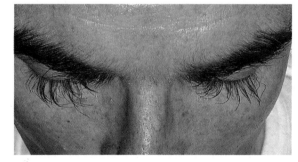

128 Elongation of the eyelashes is sometimes noted in HIV disease. This has been reported to be associated with high prolactin levels.

127 Pale nail beds, a nonspecific sign of serious illness, are often seen in HIV disease.

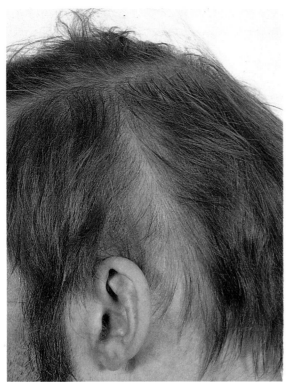

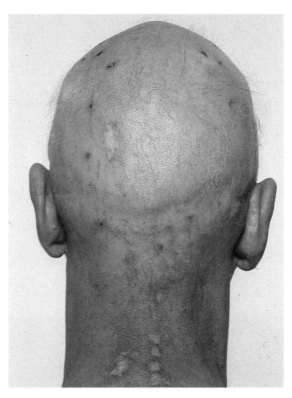

129 Diffuse alopecia is very common in advanced HIV disease.

130 Alopecia totalis in a patient with advanced ARC. Hair loss to this extent is unusual.

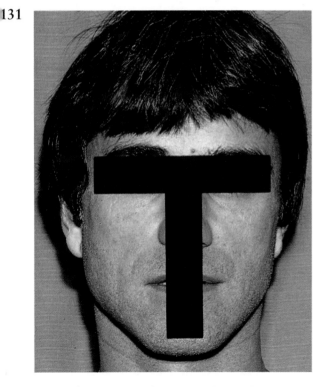

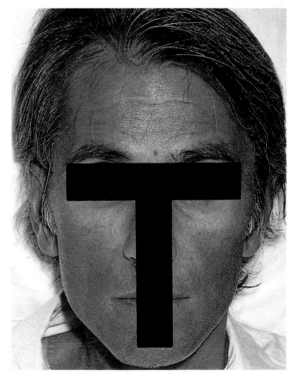

131 and **132 Rapid ageing.** These photographs were taken with an interval of two years. Premature greying, frontal recession and thinning of hair, loss of facial fat with hollowing of contours contribute to this appearance.

133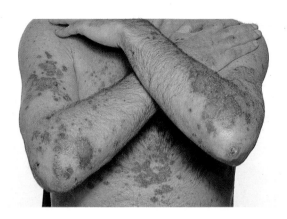

134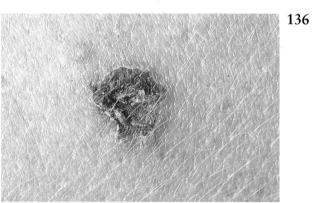

133 and **134** **Psoriasis** in patients with HIV disease. Psoriasis may present for the first time or existing psoriasis may be exacerbated with the advancing immunosuppression of HIV disease.

135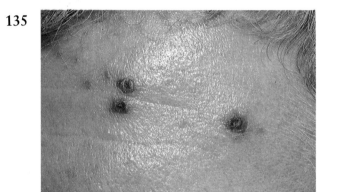

136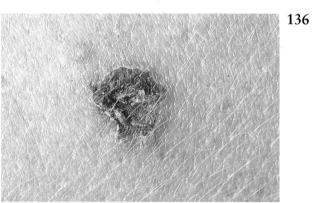

135 and **136** **Disseminated varicella zoster virus infection** in a terminally ill AIDS patient. These haemorrhagic, infarcted-looking lesions appeared repeatedly in this seriously ill patient with probable HIV encephalopathy. Varicella zoster virus was cultured from the lesions and was visible on electron microscopy (**136**). Similar lesions have been described in a patient with disseminated cutaneous cytomegalovirus infection.

137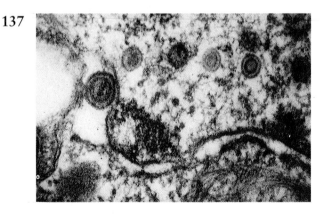

137 **Herpes virus particles** visible on electron microscopy in a skin biopsy of the patient in **134** and **135**.

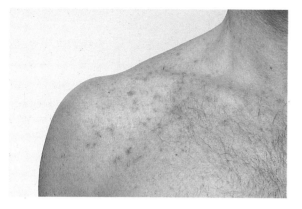

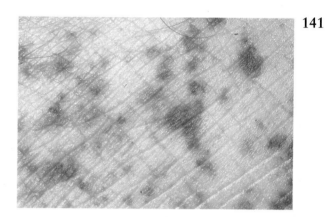

138 and 139   Grover's acantholytic dermatosis – a benign scaly eruption on the shoulder of a patient with ARC. This skin eruption seems to be more common in HIV disease.

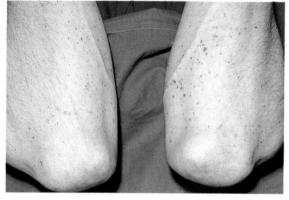

140 and 141   Cutaneous vasculitis in a patient with AIDS. Several patients have been described with an immune complex vasculitis in AIDS. This is an uncommon finding and seldom leads to systemic vasculitis.

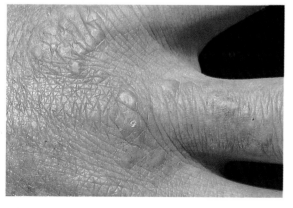

142 and 143   Granuloma annulare in a patient with ARC. There is dispute as to whether this uncommon condition is statistically more common in patients with HIV disease.

Section 14: ENT problems

Patients with HIV disease are more prone to certain infectious and allergic ENT problems and may in fact first present their HIV disease to the ear, nose and throat specialist. The following problems are seen:

1 catarrh/postnasal drip
2 sinusitis
3 otitis media
4 serous otitis media
5 otitis externa
6 nerve deafness.

The commonest problem is continuous postnasal drip. This may lead to coughing at night. It is possibly on the basis of allergic rhinitis and symptomatic relief can be obtained with the use of corticosteroid nasal sprays. Interestingly the nasal mucosa has a granular appearance. Sinusitis and otitis media are frequently due to infection with Haemophilus and the former may be so severe with fever and pain that patients may be admitted to hospital with suspected meningitis or PUO (pyrexia of unknown origin).

Serous otitis media with complaints of 'clicking in the ears like going up in an aeroplane' and sometimes middle ear deafness is very common in advanced HIV disease and may be related to weight loss in the face leading to a patulous eustachian tube which blocks allowing negative pressure and collection of secretions in the middle ear. The increased incidence of otitis externa may be secondary to the increased incidence of seborrhoeic dermatitis. Eighth nerve deafness is an occasional problem and probably a manifestation of HIV neuropathy.

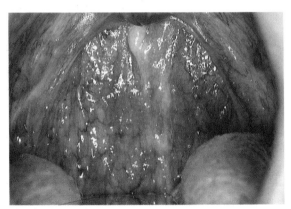

144 Serous discharge from postnasal drip seen on the posterior pharyngeal wall in a patient with AIDS.

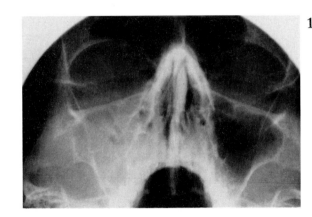

145 Opaque maxillary sinus in a patient with sinusitis admitted initially to hospital for an investigation of PUO.

Section 15: Kaposi's sarcoma

Kaposi's sarcoma was first described by the Hungarian dermatologist Moritz Kaposi (146) in 1872. He described a slowly growing usually benign tumour in elderly Italian or East European men of Jewish descent which usually presented on the lower limbs (147). Later Kaposi's sarcoma of both benign and more aggressive type was found to be widespread in Africa. In 1981 the first HIV related cases were described in the US where 35% of AIDS was found to present with this previously very rare tumour. In AIDS the distribution can be classical with lesions appearing firstly on the lower legs (153 and 154) but more commonly lesions are scattered widely over the body (148 and 149).

The cell of origin is the endothelial cell and the tumour is thought not to metastasise but to be multicentric. It is common in homosexuals with AIDS but rare in the other risk groups. The reason for this is unknown but KS may be due to an as yet unidentified 'opportunistic' sarcoma virus widespread in the homosexual community but rare in others – perhaps a virus that is spread by sexual contact but not by intravenous drug use.

Kaposi's sarcoma may be very aggressive in AIDS and death may result from pulmonary involvement. It is more usual, however, for an AIDS patient with Kaposi's sarcoma to die of an opportunistic infection or encephalopathy rather than of the tumour itself. Widespead involvement of the gastrointestinal tract occurs (see Section 18) but cerebral involvement is exceedingly rare.

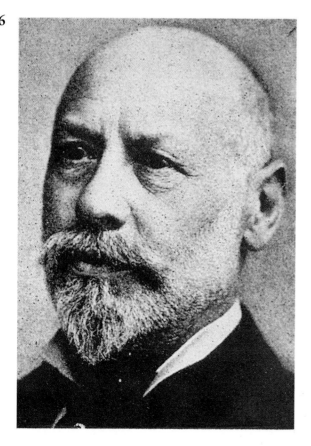

146   Moritz Kaposi.

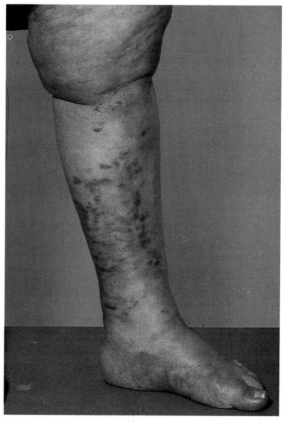

147   Classical Kaposi's sarcoma in an elderly Jewish man.

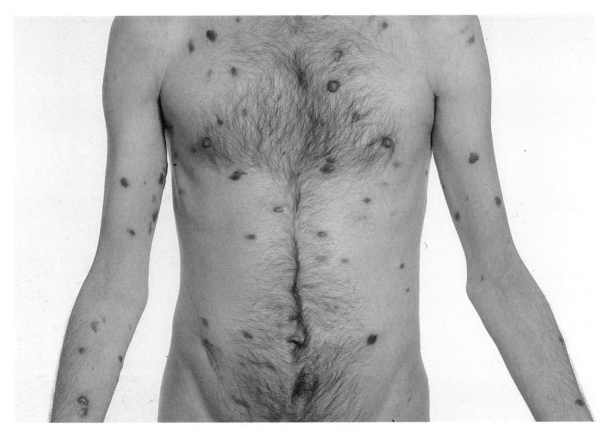

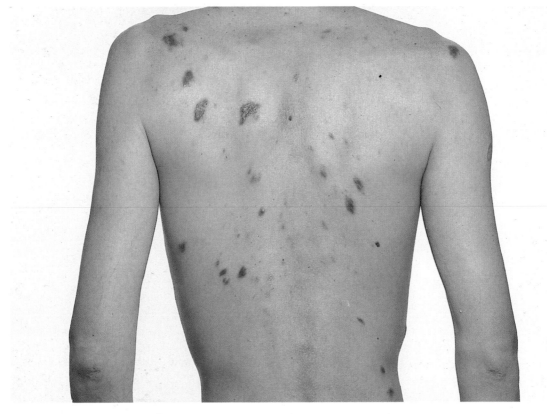

148 and **149**   Kaposi's sarcoma: Widespread lesions in two different patients with AIDS.

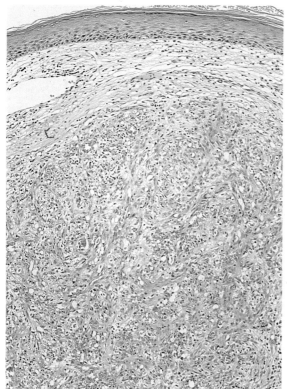

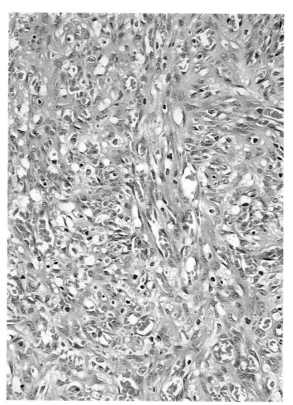

150 Histopathology of a Kaposi's sarcoma nodule in the skin (H&E × 25). With normal dermis overlying it, the tumour nodule can be seen to consist of a mass of spindle cells with many red blood cells in vascular spaces and haemosiderin deposition.

151 Higher magnification of 150 showing poorly formed vascular channels within the tumour formed by the atypical endothelial cells. There are increased mitoses to be seen but the tumour does not look particularly malignant. Lesions may be misdiagnosed as benign angiomas and if Kaposi's sarcoma is suspected clinically the histopathologist should always be informed.

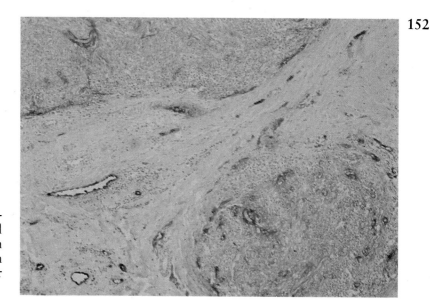

152 Immunocytochemical staining for Factor VIII. Both endothelial and Kaposi's sarcoma cells stain positive for Factor VIII (dark brown staining) — evidence that the tumour cells are of endothelial origin.

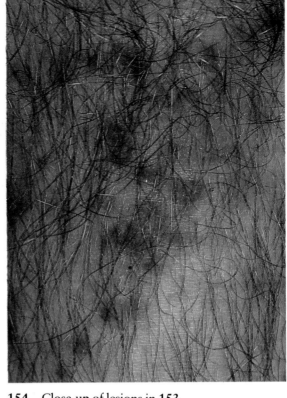

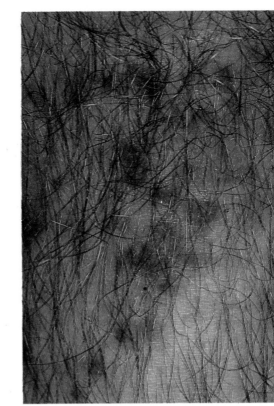

153   Kaposi's sarcoma presenting on the lower leg in a patient with AIDS – as in classical Kaposi's sarcoma. About a third of AIDS Kaposi's sarcoma presents on the lower legs.

154   Close-up of lesions in **153**.

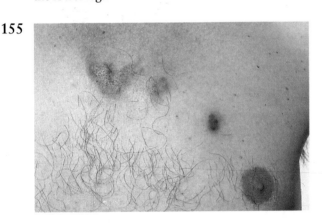

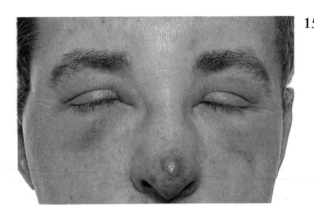

155   Kaposi's sarcoma lesions are often surrounded by bruising and oedema, particularly in dependent areas. This is perhaps not surprising when it is considered that the tumour is a mesh of poorly formed 'leaky' blood vessels (see **150** and **151**).

156   Periorbital oedema in a patient with advanced Kaposi's sarcoma. Oedema of the face, particularly around the eyes, is common when Kaposi's sarcoma involves the face and in severe cases it leads to closure of the eyes. Ankle oedema (**185**) and scrotal oedema (**187**) also occur.

157 **158** **159**

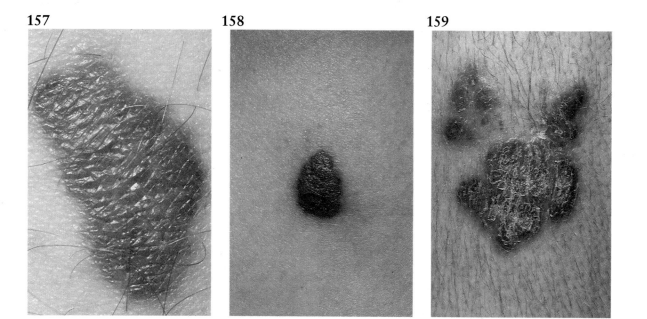

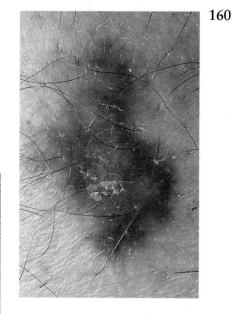
160

157 to **160** **Kaposi's sarcoma lesions** from different patients to show variation in colour and appearance. Older lesions are darker and may become scaly (**159**).

161 **162**

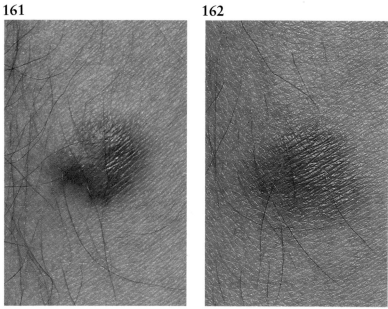

161 and **162** **Kaposi lesions** may sometimes spontaneously regress as in this case. Although the lesion may flatten, however, haemosiderin staining usually remains.

163

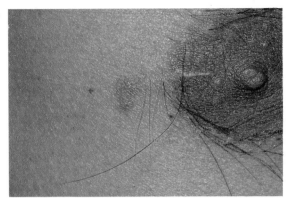

163 and 164   Early lesions of Kaposi's sarcoma. At this stage the lesions are entirely macular and impalpable.

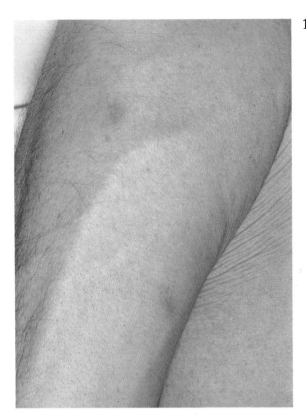

165

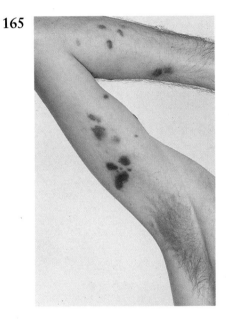

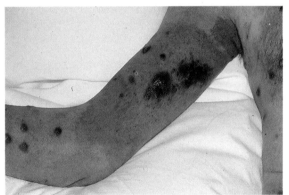

165 and 166   Kaposi's sarcoma lesions progressing with time on the arm of a patient with advanced disease. In **166** the nodular lesions can be seen to be surrounded by what looks like purpura. This appearance is actually due to infiltration of the whole skin by the tumour giving the arm a woody and indurated feel like lymphoedema.

167

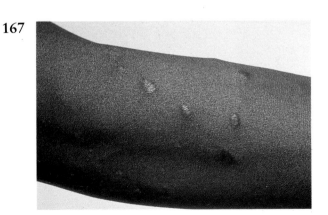

167   Disseminated Kaposi's sarcoma in an African patient with AIDS. In Africa aggressive Kaposi's sarcoma is found usually to be HIV antibody positive. Benign Kaposi's sarcoma is usually HIV antibody negative and unrelated to AIDS.

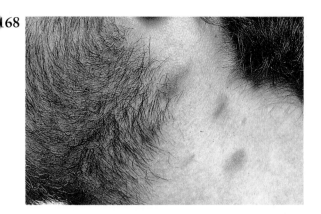

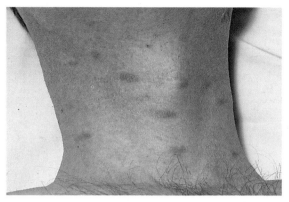

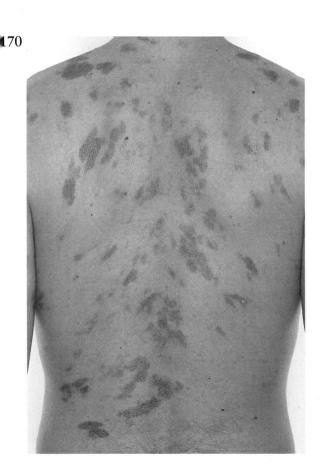

168 to **170**   A special feature of Kaposi's sarcoma lesions is that they may line up along skin creases as can be seen in the neck in these two patients and from the 'Christmas tree effect' on the back of the third patient.

Kaposi's sarcoma – common sites

171 to 174 Kaposi's sarcoma in the mouth. Kaposi's sarcoma frequently involves the hard palate and the area first involved is usually above the second molar tooth. In **172** and **173** these were the first Kaposi lesions seen in these two patients. The lesions on the palate are usually macular but may be raised as in **173** and **174**.

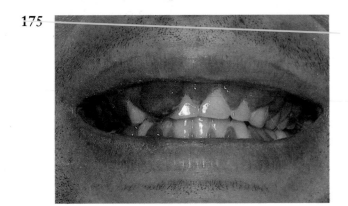

175 Aggressive Kaposi's sarcoma may involve the gingival margin. This makes dental hygiene particularly difficult and especially important.

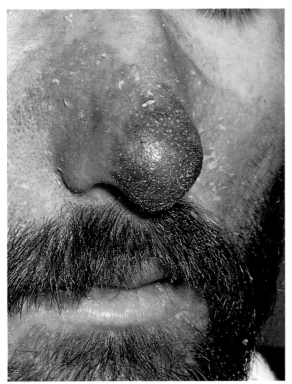

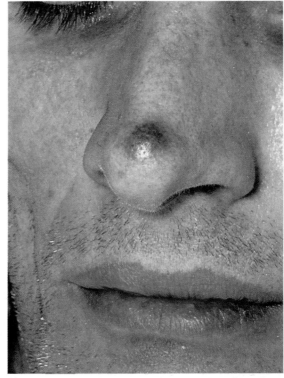

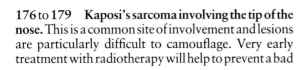

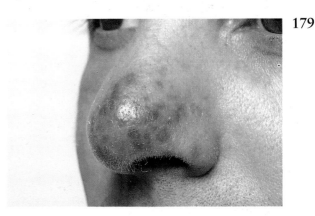

176 to 179   Kaposi's sarcoma involving the tip of the nose. This is a common site of involvement and lesions are particularly difficult to camouflage. Very early treatment with radiotherapy will help to prevent a bad lesion, such as in **176**, developing. Laser therapy may reduce the intensity of the colour in a developed lesion. Note the seborrhoeic dermatitis in a butterfly distribution on the face in **176**.

180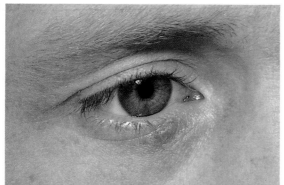

180 Kaposi's sarcoma lesion at the junction of the medial third and lateral two thirds of the **lower eyelid.**

181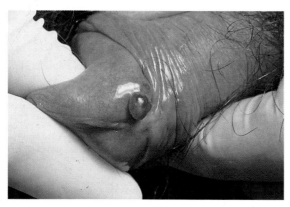

182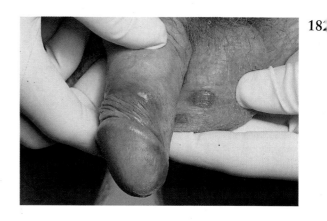

181 and 182 Kaposi's sarcoma lesions on the **penis.**

183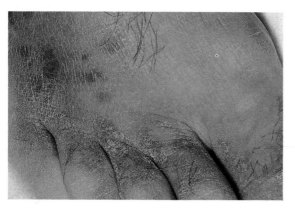

184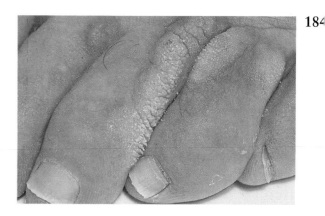

183 and 184 Kaposi's sarcoma lesions of the **toes**—a common site with varied appearance, **183** resembling bruising and **184** showing the warty presentation that may sometimes occur.

Treatment options in Kaposi's sarcoma

Kaposi's sarcoma may be treated locally by excision, radiotherapy or intralesional chemotherapy, or systemically with alpha interferon or chemotherapy. The choice of therapy is determined by the size and quantity of the lesions, and their site. The aim of treatment is usually to improve or prevent deterioration in cosmetic appearance to give relief from locally troublesome oedematous or painful lesions.

Overall prognosis is probably little affected by treatment except in some cases of aggressive Kaposi's sarcoma, perhaps with pulmonary involvement, when survival is likely to be prolonged if a partial remission is achieved. The tumour is very susceptible to radiother-apy and chemotherapy and the low dose single agent systemic chemotherapy regimes that are usually administered (with agents such as vinblastine, vincristine, bleomycin or VP16) probably seldom add to the degree of immunosuppression.

High dose conventional chemotherapy regimes are immunosuppressive, however, and may worsen prognosis by causing more rapid development of major opportunistic infections. Alpha interferon, while not immunosuppressive, is generally less well tolerated than chemotherapy with unpleasant side effects of fever and flu-like symptoms. It is also extremely expensive.

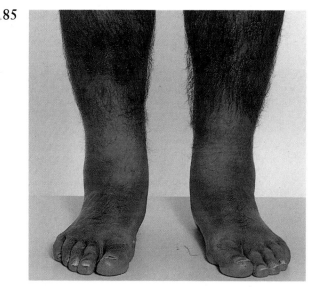

185 Kaposi's sarcoma of the lower legs with oedema. These lesions were tender and painful.

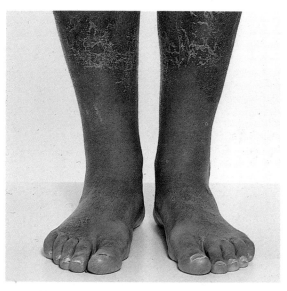

186 Same patient as in **185** with resolution of oedema and pain after radiotherapy to shins. Note also the loss of hair. During radiotherapy treatment lesions may swell and temporarily become more tender, therefore early treatment is recommended for lesions on the shin and the soles of the feet which often become tender with time.

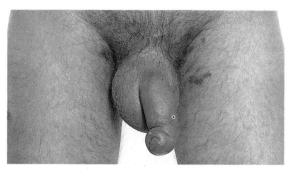

187 Oedema of the genitalia in a patient with Kaposi's sarcoma involving inguinal glands.

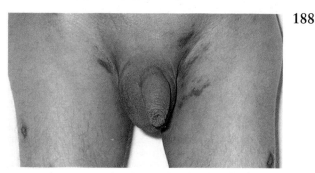

188 Resolution of oedema after local radiotherapy treatment.

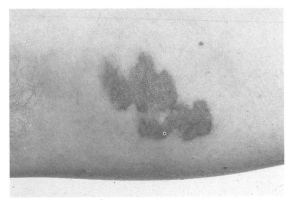

189 Kaposi's sarcoma lesion on the arm.

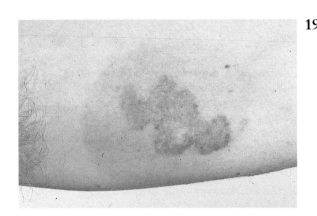

190 Same lesion as in **189** after treatment with local radiotherapy. Note that the lesion has flattened (and stopped growing) but haemosiderin staining remains. Note also the surrounding pigmentation from the radiotherapy beam. This will fade with time and is less of a problem if well-fractionated treatment is given rather than single dose radiotherapy.

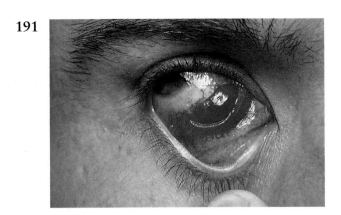

191 Kaposi's sarcoma lesion of the conjunctiva.

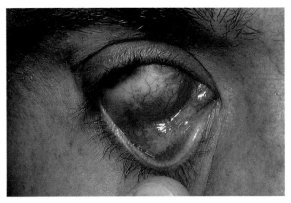

192 Resolution of lesion in **191** after local radiotherapy.

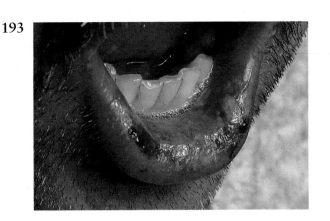

193 **Severe mucositis** in a patient who had received local radiotherapy to the gingiva for Kaposi's sarcoma. AIDS patients are particularly susceptible to mucositis when radiotherapy is used in the mouth and it is probably best avoided – systemic chemotherapy being used instead. If radiotherapy is used in the mouth it should be low dose and well-fractionated.

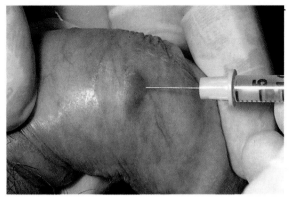

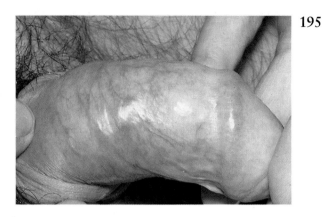

194 Small Kaposi's sarcoma lesion on the penis being treated with intralesional chemotherapy with vinblastine 0.2 mg/ml. This form of treatment is best reserved for lesions under 1 cm and will often result in arrest of growth or resolution of the lesion. 0.1-0.2 ml is injected in the centre of the lesion and the treatment may have to be repeated several times.

195 Resolution of Karposi's sarcoma lesion on the penis after intralesional chemotherapy.

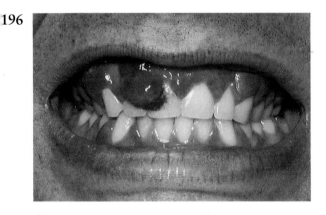

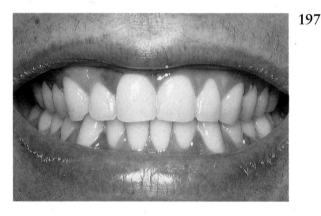

196 Severe gingival involvement with Kaposi's sarcoma.

197 Resolution of Kaposi's sarcoma in the patient in 196 after treatment with systemic VP16.

198

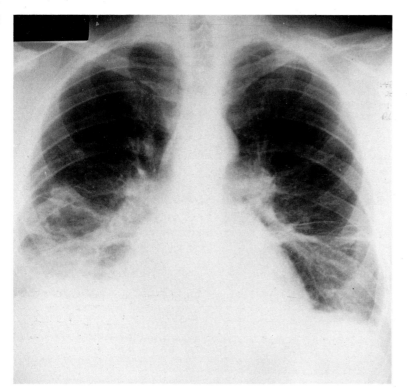

198 Marked pulmonary involvement with Kaposi's sarcoma and probable pleural effusion. This patient was breathless.

199

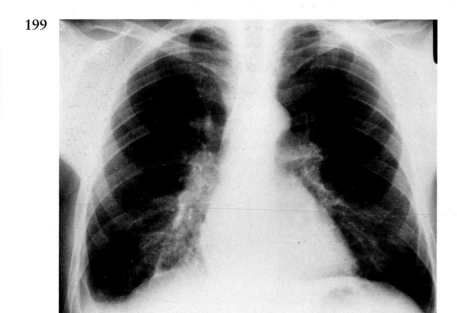

199 Same patient as in 198 one month later after weekly treatments with vincristine and bleomycin. The patient's breathlessness had resolved. Kaposi lung is a particularly aggressive and unpleasant complication and often does not respond to treatment.

Section 16: Pulmonary disease

Some 60% of 'AIDS' presents with pneumonia, the vast majority of which is caused by the protozoan *Pneumocystis carinii*. A typical patient presents with a persistent nonproductive dry cough of some weeks' duration (which comes in paroxysms and may lead to vomiting), fever, and exertional dyspnoea. The most important clinical sign is tachypnoea at rest. Other clinical signs in the chest are usually absent. A blood gas analysis may show hypoxia and a chest x-ray may show bilateral interstitial shadowing. However, any or all of these investigations may be normal.

Fibreoptic bronchoscopy (see 260) with alveolar lavage or transbronchial biopsy is usually required to establish the diagnosis although occasionally sputum induced by hypertonic saline inhalation may contain pneumocysts.

The early diagnosis of *Pneumocystis carinii* pneumonia (PCP) is of vital importance. The onset is often subtle and the patient may feel and look quite well. Dry cough and particularly shortness of breath should never be lightly dismissed in an HIV antibody positive person even if a chest x-ray and blood gas analysis are initially normal.

If treatment is initiated before there are chest x-ray signs the chances of survival are high (>80%) but if treatment is delayed (perhaps because the patient is initially turned away from hospital with false reassurance) and the patient is significantly hypoxic when treatment begins, the survival rate is much worse (approximately 50%). The treatment of choice is co-trimoxazole in high dose intravenously. Alternative treatments are pentamidine intravenously or by inhalation, trimethoprim/dapsone, efflornithine and trimotrexate. Treatment should be started on clinical suspicion and not necessarily delayed until substantive proof of the diagnosis, otherwise vital time may be lost.

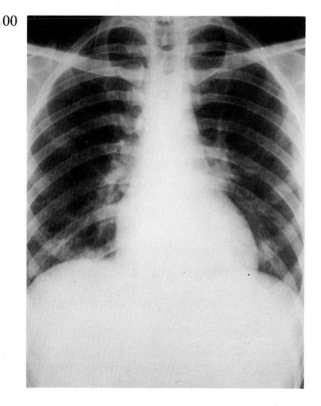

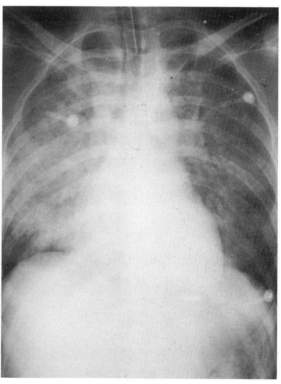

200 ***Pneumocystis carinii* pneumonia (PCP) on presentation.** Although the chest x-ray shows little shadowing, the patient was markedly hypoxic on admission and a transbronchial biopsy revealed *Pneumocystis carinii*.

201 The same patient shown in 200 four days later showing rapid deterioration. This patient died despite high dose intravenous co-trimoxazole – the treatment of choice.

Many other chest infections occur in HIV disease. However, by far the most common is PCP. Some of the other chest infections that occur in HIV disease are CMV pneumonitis, tuberculosis and pneumococcal lobar pneumonia. Mixed infections are common.

All patients who have suffered PCP, and perhaps those with a low CD4 positive lymphocyte count, below 200/mm^3, should receive some continuous prophylaxis against PCP. The most effective prophylaxis is continuous low dose co-trimoxazole. However, this may not be tolerated and alternatives such as sulphonamide/diamino-pyrimidine once weekly or inhaled pentamidine fortnightly are also effective.

202

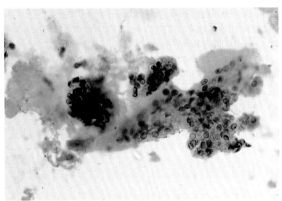

202 Cytological preparation of numerous *Pneumocystis carinii* from bronchial washings (silver methenamine – Grocott ×160).

20

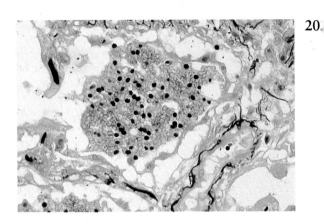

203 *Pneumocystis carinii.* Transbronchial biopsy of lung stained by Grocott method to show *Pneumocystis carinii* in the intra-alveolar exudate (Grocott ×100).

204

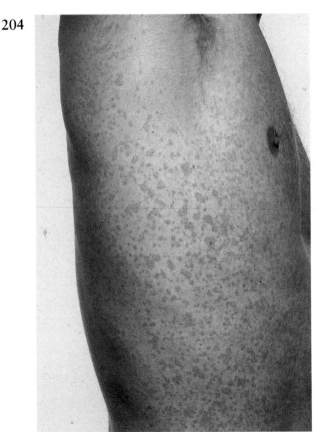

204 Co-trimoxazole rash in a patient with *Pneumocystis carinii.* Hypersensitivity to co-trimoxazole is very common in AIDS patients and occurs in 50 to 60%. A febrile reaction is also common. If the reaction is mild it may be possible to continue the co-trimoxazole covering the patient with an antihistamine such as terfenadine. If severe, an alternative treatment such as pentamidine should be substituted.

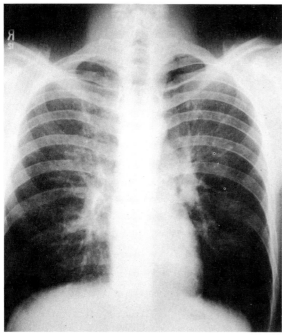

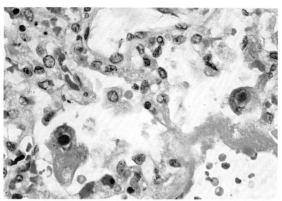

206 CMV inclusion bodies in the alveolar wall on transbronchial biopsy (H&E × 160). Documentation of CMV infection is more difficult than with PCP. Detection of CMV by DEAF test (Detection of Early Antigen by Fluorescence) is often achieved but a positive result with this test does not necessarily mean that the CMV is causing the pneumonia. CMV inclusion bodies constitute hard evidence of pathogenicity but, unfortunately, are rarely seen on biopsy specimens.

205 CMV pneumonitis, the next most common pulmonary pathogen in AIDS. The clinical presentation is indistinguishable from PCP and mixed infections often occur. Treatment is possible with ganciclovir or phosphonoformate. In a mixed infection treatment of the PCP alone often results in recovery.

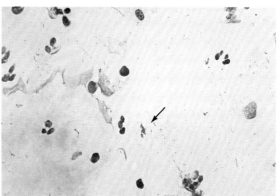

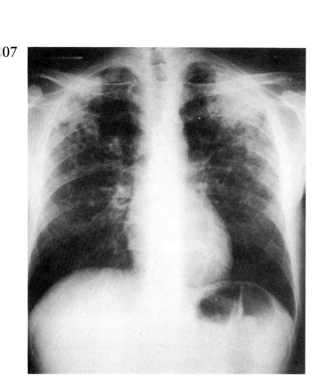

208 Sputum showing acid fast organisms (Ziehl-Neelson stain) amidst leucocytes (×160). Patients with PCP and CMV pneumonitis usually do not produce sputum but those with tuberculosis usually have a productive cough and a diagnosis may well be made by investigation of the sputum. *M. tuberculosis* usually responds promptly to conventional antituberculous agents. Atypical mycobacteria are usually highly resistant to antituberculous drugs, even to those drugs to which they may show *in vitro* sensitivity, such as ansamycin or clofazimine.

207 HIV positive patient with pulmonary tuberculosis. Frequently the clue is upper lobe shadowing as in this patient. *M. tuberculosis* in the chest does not define the patient as having AIDS, but atypical mycobacterial chest infection does.

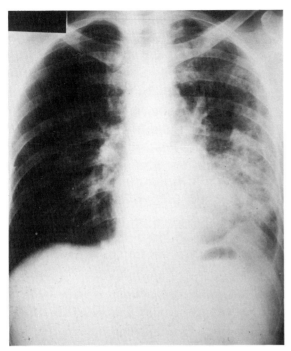

209 Patient with toxoplasma pneumonia, a rare opportunist infection in the lung even in AIDS.

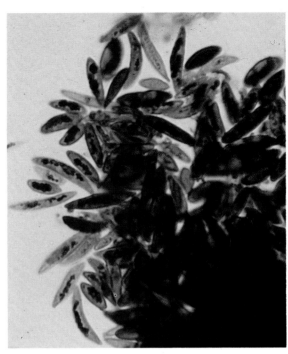

210 The same patient as in **209** showing toxoplasma trophozoites on transbronchial biopsy (Grocott ×400).

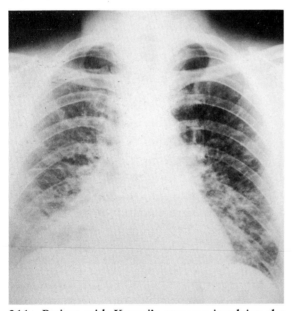

211 Patient with Kaposi's sarcoma involving the lung. Note that the interstitial shadowing is similar to that seen in PCP and CMV pneumonitis but slightly more nodular. The two can usually be distinguished clinically. The patient with Kaposi lung will usually have Kaposi lesions on the skin and will be afebrile. The patient with PCP will usually have a fever. A pleural effusion (which if tapped is blood stained) is strongly suggestive of Kaposi lung. Endobronchial haemorrhagic KS lesions can usually be seen on bronchoscopy.

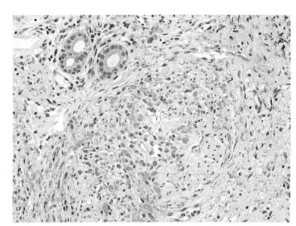

21

212 Bronchial biopsy showing Kaposi's sarcoma (H&E ×60). Note the multiple irregularly-shaped vascular spaces lined by pleomophic endothelial cells with extravasated erythrocytes (see also **151**). The prognosis for Kaposi lung is grave but there may sometimes be improvement with systemic chemotherapy (**198** and **199**). The patients may do poorly with radiotherapy to the lung fields.

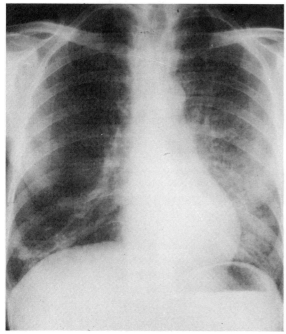

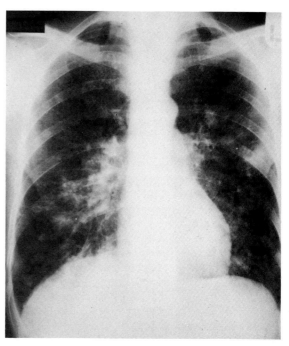

213 Interstitial shadowing in both lung fields in a patient with *Pneumocystis carinii* pneumonia.

214 Same patient as in **213** seven months after successful treatment of PCP but now with the development of Kaposi lung. Note the different appearance of the pulmonary shadowing in these two conditions.

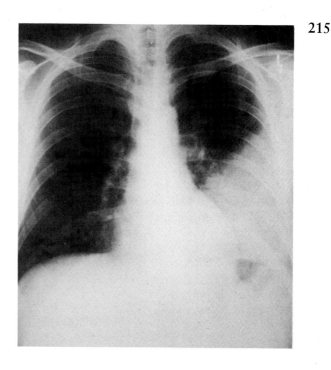

215 Patient with pneumococcal lobar pneumonia. Lobar pneumonia due to *Pneumococcus* and *Haemophilus* appears to be more common in HIV disease.

Section 17: Diseases of the nervous system

The neurology of AIDS is complex. HIV may cause damage to the nervous system directly (HIV encephalopathy) or indirectly with opportunistic infections secondary to immunosuppression.

1 HIV encephalopathy/myelopathy/peripheral nerve lesions. Some two thirds of patients with AIDS are said to suffer from HIV encephalopathy. This has been called the AIDS dementia complex but the term is somewhat misleading as usually dementia is very subtle with only mild short term memory loss and personality change, except in very ill preterminal patients. If the spinal cord is involved, ataxia, incontinence and paraplegia may be part of the clinical picture. An initial flaccid paralysis of the legs may become spastic. Speech may be slurred. Peripheral nerve lesions, particularly foot drop, and epileptic fits may occur. HIV encephalopathy is a manifestation of late stage HIV disease and usually occurs in AIDS patients after one or more opportunistic infections. HIV encephalopathy should be a diagnosis of exclusion as memory loss and personality change can be caused by many other secondary CNS problems in HIV disease, such as cerebral abscess or tumour, and a CT scan or nuclear magnetic resonance (NMR) scan should be performed to exclude these possibilities. Two viral opportunistic infections — progressive multifocal leucoencephalopathy and cytomegalovirus encephalitis — may also mimic HIV encephalopathy.

2 Focal lesions, which most commonly present with either focal paralysis or fits, are most likely to be due to cerebral toxoplasmosis. In most units a focal lesion on the CT scan in an HIV antibody positive patient is treated as cerebral toxoplasmosis to see if there is clinical improvement before brain biopsy is performed. The second most likely cause of an intracerebral mass in HIV disease is a CNS lymphoma. Other much rarer possibilities are tuberculoma or fungal abscess.

3 Meningitis. The commonest cause of meningitis in a patient with AIDS is *Cryptococcus* and the second commonest cause is mycobacteria. Presentation may be very subtle, the patient complaining of headache and appearing slightly vague. This may persist for some days or weeks. There may be no photophobia or neck stiffness and on lumbar puncture there may be no inflammatory cells seen. Special stains should always be used, however, to detect *Cryptococcus* or mycobacteria which may be found in the absence of an inflammatory response. Bacterial meningitis does not seem common in HIV disease.

4 Retinitis. Cytomegalovirus retinitis is a common cause of blindness in HIV disease. The patient may present complaining either of blurry vision, pain in the eye, or visual field defect. Fundoscopic appearance is distinctive (see **225** and **226**). Treatment should be instituted urgently with an anti-CMV drug such as ganciclovir or phosphonoformate in an attempt to preserve sight.

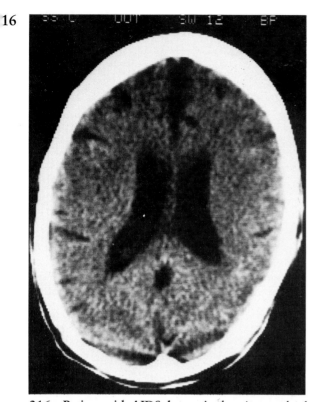

216 **Patient with AIDS dementia** showing cerebral atrophy with enlarged lateral ventricles on CT scan.

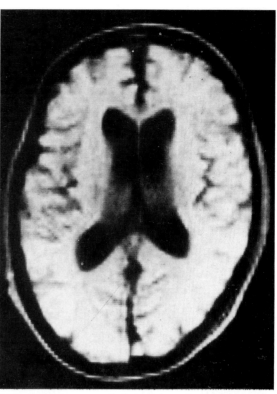

217 NMR scan of the patient in **216** showing shrunken cerebral hemispheres.

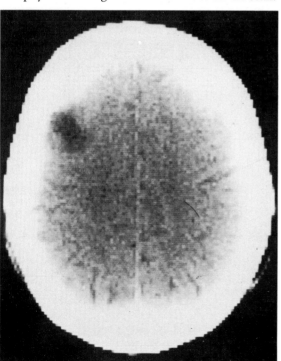

218 CT scan of a patient with toxoplasma cerebral abscess.

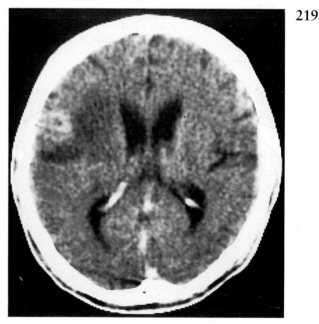

219 CT scan of the brain of a patient with AIDS showing a cerebral lymphoma in the left cerebral hemisphere with surrounding cerebral oedema.

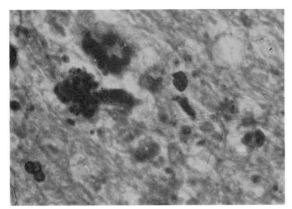

220 Histopathology of a brain at post mortem showing cerebral toxoplasmosis.

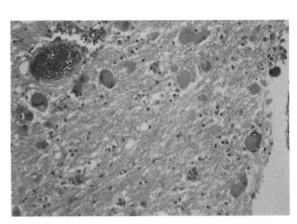

221 Histopathology of the brain at post mortem of a patient who died from CMV encephalitis. Multiple CMV inclusion bodies can be seen. It is difficult to document this infection in life, the acute encephalitic picture being similar to that of HIV encephalopathy.

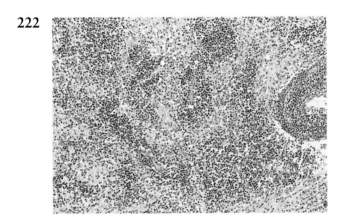

222 Brain from a patient with AIDS showing **microgliomatosis**, a form of malignant lymphoma (H&E ×25). Some evidence suggests that Epstein-Barr virus is a cause of CNS lymphoma in AIDS.

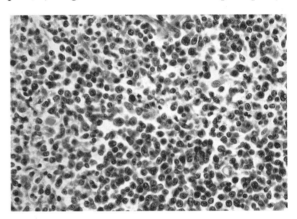

223 Higher power of **222**. Sheets of intermediate-sized cells having clefted nuclei, conspicuous nucleoli and fairly numerous mitotic figures (H&E × 100).

224 A

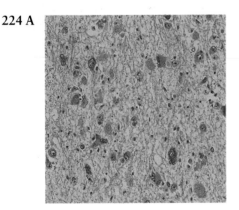

224 B

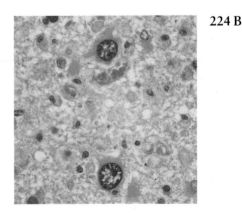

224 A and B Histopathology of the brain of an AIDS patient showing destruction from progressive multi-focal leucoencephalopathy. Note destruction of the white matter. This infection caused by parvovirus SV40 often results in focal lesions and fits and may have a very rapid course.

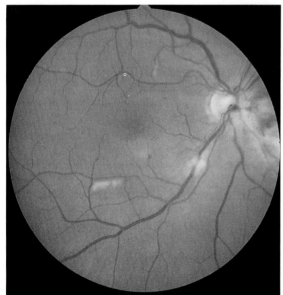

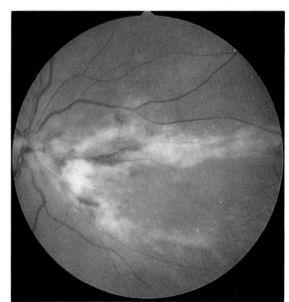

225 and 226 CMV retinitis in patient with AIDS.
This serious opportunistic infection can rapidly
progress to irreversible blindness. CMV causes a
retinal vasculitis which leads to areas of infarction.
Treatment is possible with ganciclovir or phosphonoformate and maintenance therapy is usually required
to prevent reactivation.

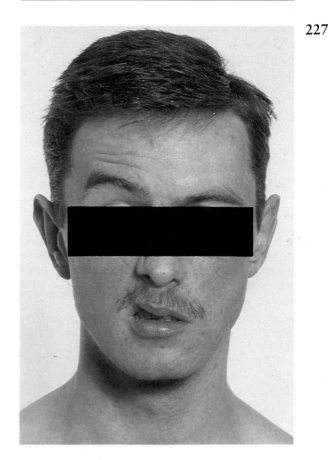

**227 Left sided facial nerve palsy (Bell's palsy) in a
patient with AIDS.** This occasional problem recovers
spontaneously. The cause is uncertain but it may be
related to shingles involving the facial nerve and
should probably be treated with high dose acyclovir.

Section 18: Gastrointestinal disease

HIV disease may present in the gastrointestinal system with diarrhoea, oesophagitis, progressive anal herpes or Kaposi's sarcoma of the gut.

Diarrhoea

1 Cryptosporidium

Cryptosporidium is a protozoal organism that was not realised to be a pathogen in man before it was discovered to be causing disease in AIDS patients. It is now recognised as a common cause of travellers' diarrhoea resulting in a one or two week illness in the nonimmunocompromised host. In AIDS it can cause a severe chronic, even fatal, diarrhoea. It is important when investigating diarrhoea in HIV antibody positive patients to look specifically for this parasite which is only visible with special stains, such as acid fast. Cryptosporidial diarrhoea may be treated with erythromycin or spyromycin. The response is often only partial and it is unusual to clear the organism. Cryptosporidial diarrhoea persisting for over a month satisfies the CDC criteria for AIDS (see Appendix A).

2 Cytomegalovirus (CMV)

CMV causes a chronic diarrhoea often associated with abdominal pain and signs of peritonism. Rectal biopsy may reveal diagnostic inclusion bodies (**232**) but may often be negative. A relatively deep biopsy is required to show inclusion bodies. CMV diarrhoea may be associated with CMV oesophagitis, retinitis, or pneumonitis. Treatment with ganciclovir or phosphonoformate may be successful but again maintenance therapy is usually required. The prognosis is very poor.

3 Atypical mycobacteria

Atypical mycobacteria (especially *Mycobacterium avium intracellulare* (MAI)) may involve the gastrointestinal tract extensively, producing a Whipple's-like syndrome. It is most easily cultured from the stool or blood and may be seen on acid fast stain of the stool (**234**). In a patient with a PUO in whom MAI is not visible in the stool, liver biopsy may reveal the organism on acid fast stain before culture results are available (**235**). Disseminated MAI satisfies the CDC criteria for AIDS.

4 Giardiasis

Giardia is a common cause of diarrhoea in HIV positive patients. It usually responds to metronidazole but may require a longer course than for the nonimmunocompromised patient. Although a common problem, giardiasis does not satisfy the CDC criteria for AIDS.

5 Salmonella

Salmonella typhimurium, an intracellular bacterial gut pathogen, is another common cause of diarrhoea in patients with HIV disease. Recurrent salmonella septicaemia satisfies the CDC criteria for AIDS.

6 Campylobacter

Campylobacter is another organism that seems to cause diarrhoea not infrequently in patients with ARC and AIDS. It responds to erythromycin.

228

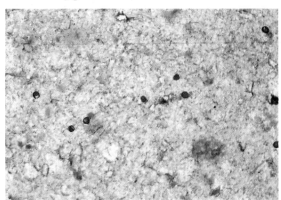

228   *Cryptosporidium* in a stool from a patient with diarrhoea (Ziehl-Neelsen ×160).

229

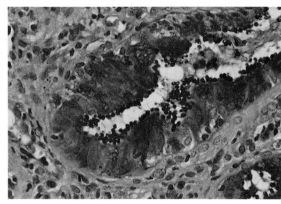

229   Periodic acid Shiff preparation of rectal biopsy (×100) showing crypt lined by numerous *Cryptosporidia* stained dark magenta.

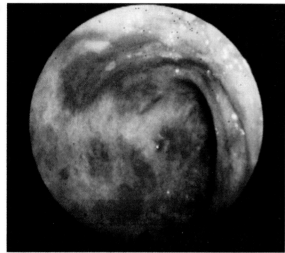

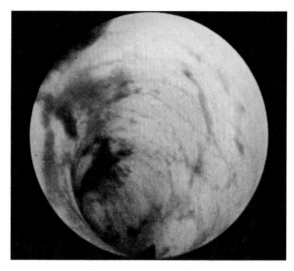

230 Colonoscopy showing inflammation in a patient with CMV colitis.

231 Repeat colonoscopy in the patient in 230 showing resolution of inflammation after treatment with ganciclovir.

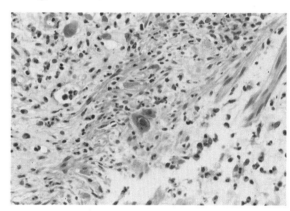

232 Cytomegalic inclusion body in the rectal mucosa of a patient with cytomegalovirus enterocolitis. Note the body surrounded by a clear halo and the nuclear membrane (H&E ×120).

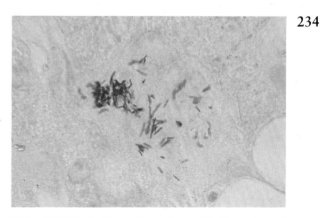

233 *Mycobacterium avium intracellulare* in stool (Ziehl-Neelsen ×160).

234 MAI in the liver of a patient with disseminated mycobacterial infection.

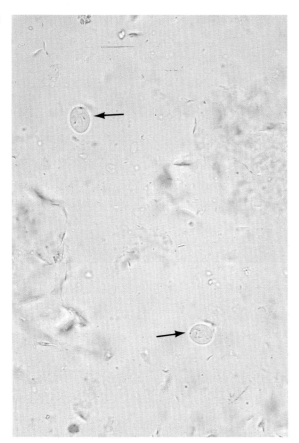

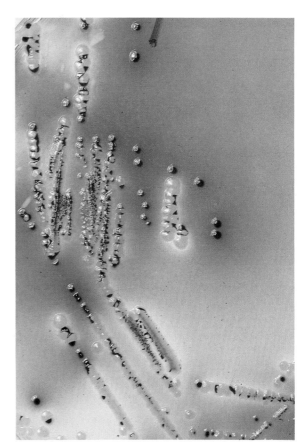

235 *Giardia lamblia* in the stool of a patient with ARC. (Wet preparation ×160.)

236 *Salmonella typhimurium* culture growing from the stool of a patient with ARC and gastroenteritis (XLD agar). Note yellow lactose fermenting colonies of *E. coli* and colourless colonies of salmonella with black centres and pink haloes.

Oesophagitis

The commonest cause of oesophagitis resulting in dysphagia in a patient with AIDS is *Candida*. This is nearly always associated with oral thrush and responds well to treatment by ketoconazole. Herpes simplex and cytomegalovirus may also result in oesophagitis – the latter often causing linear ulcers at the lower end of the oesophagus which persist for long periods. Treatment with ganciclovir or phosphono-formate may result in healing.

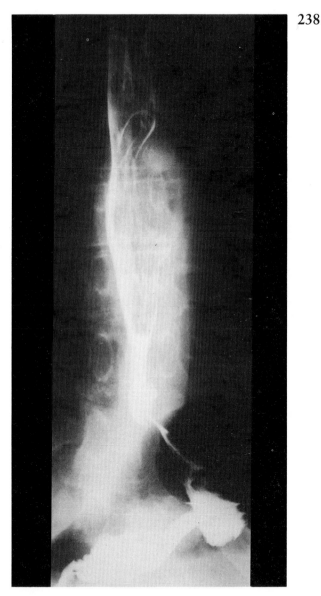

237 Candidal oesophagitis (barium swallow). Ulceration can be seen on the whole length of the oesophagus. When *Candida* involves the oesophagus it satisfies the CDC criteria for AIDS.

238 Herpes simplex oesophagitis (barium swallow). This patient had a particularly painful dysphagia which responded promptly to intravenous acyclovir.

239

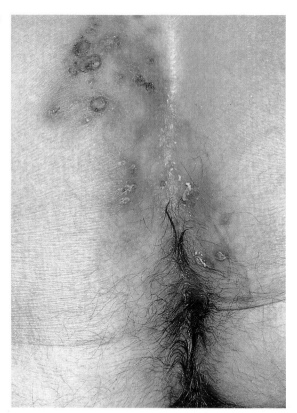

Anal herpes

239, 240 Progressive perianal herpes simplex.
Herpes simplex of the anus is an extremely common
problem in patients with HIV disease and, if persisting
for a month, satisfies the CDC criteria for AIDS. Very
often only a tiny ulcer or fissure is seen yet the patient
may be in great discomfort. Treatment with oral
acyclovir should not be delayed in patients with
painful perianal lesions.

240

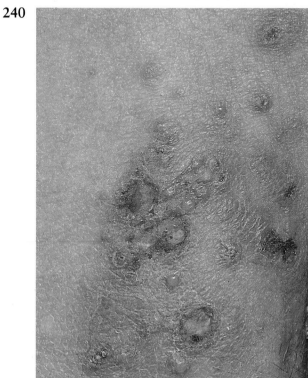

Kaposi's sarcoma of the gastrointestinal tract

Kaposi's sarcoma frequently involves the gastrointestinal tract but it is usually asymptomatic. Lesions on the hard palate are common and may be the site of presentation (**172** and **173**). Lesions may also be seen on the posterior pharyngeal wall, in the stomach and in the rectum (**244** and **245**). In the stomach wall the lesions are often painful and may be found to be the only cause of a patient's upper abdominal discomfort.

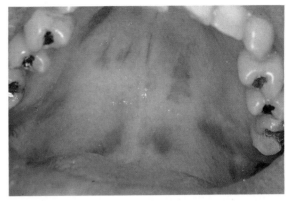

241

241 **Kaposi's sarcoma of the palate** in a patient with AIDS.

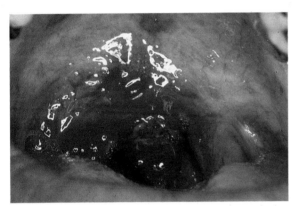

242 **Kaposi's sarcoma involving the soft palate and uvula** in a patient with AIDS.

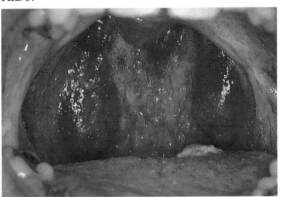

243

243 **Kaposi's sarcoma involving the posterior pharyngeal wall** in a patient with AIDS.

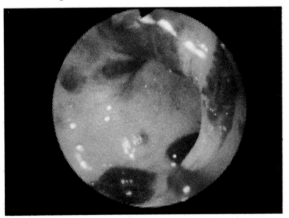

244 **Kaposi's sarcoma of the rectum** on colonoscopy.

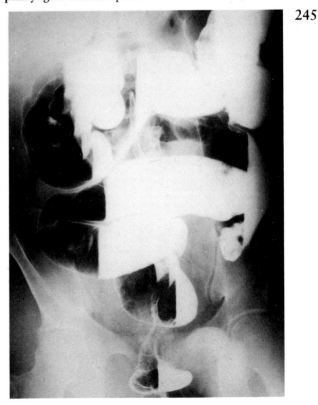

245

245 Obstruction in the rectum secondary to Kaposi's sarcoma (barium enema).

Section 19: Lymphoma

The lymphoma of AIDS is usually of non-Hodgkin's type. It usually responds to conventional chemotherapy but the bone marrow is unusually susceptible to cytotoxic drugs, and the amount of treatment that can be given may be limited.

Patients with disease limited to one anatomical site tend to do well with treatment. Those with disseminated lymphoma tend to do poorly.

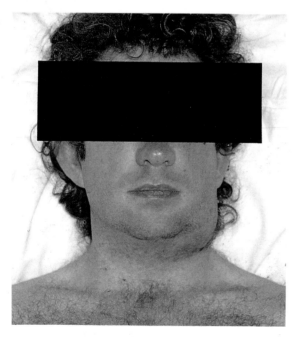

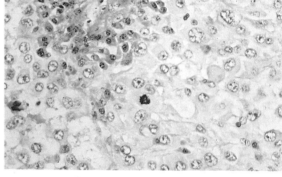

246   Posterior cervical lymph node enlarged secondary to lymphoma in a patient with AIDS.

247   Lymph node biopsy from the patient in **246**, showing non-Hodgkin's high grade histiocytic lymphoma (H&E ×100).

248   Enlarged anterior cervical nodes in a patient with lymphoma.

249   Lymph node biopsy from the patient in **248** showing poorly-differentiated diffuse non-Hodgkin's malignant lymphoma of small and intermediate cell type.

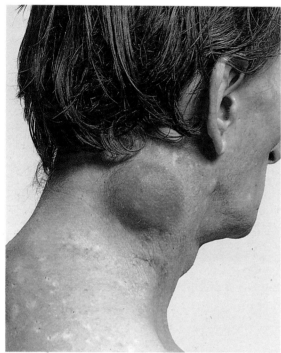

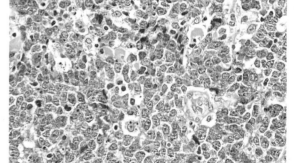

Section 20: Paediatric HIV disease

HIV disease in children shows significant differences from the disease in adults. The incubation period is usually shorter. Children fail to thrive and retarded cerebral development results in failure to achieve milestones. Gram negative septicaemia is common in children with HIV disease but not adults. Also two clinical entities rarely seen in adults occur—lymphocytic interstitial pneumonitis (LIP), probably due to Epstein-Barr infection of the lung (250), and chronic parotid swelling, the cause of which is uncertain (251 and 252). An abnormal facial development has also been described in children with HIV disease (253). Because of the many differences between adult and paediatric HIV disease a separate classification of paediatric disease has been drawn up by the Center for Disease Control (CDC). Because of difficulty in establishing whether a child under 15 months is truly HIV infected or HIV antibody positive because of passive transfer of maternal immunoglobulins during pregnancy, a separate definition of HIV disease for those under 15 months has been drawn up by the CDC.

250 Chest x-ray of a young child who is asymptomatic with lymphocytic interstitial pneumonitis (LIP). Note the reticular pattern unlike the diffuse pattern seen with PCP.

PCP and LIP can usually be distinguished on clinical grounds. Although both conditions may cause breathlessness, patients with PCP suffer an acute illness with fever whereas LIP results in a chronic condition without fever. Improvement in LIP after steroid treatment has been reported, but this is controversial.

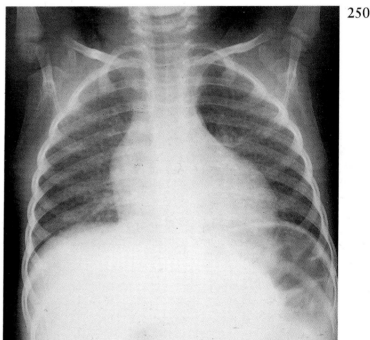

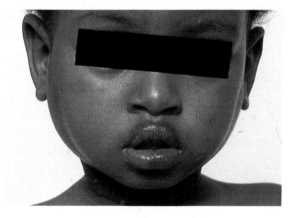
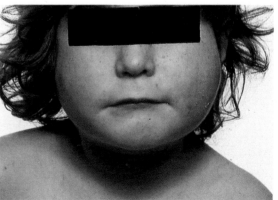

251 and 252 Bilateral parotid swelling in two little girls with HIV disease. Cause unknown.

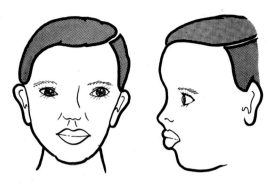

253 Diagram showing the dysmorphic facial features that have been described with congenital HIV infection. A flat nasal bridge with a prominent forehead, patulous lips with a triangular philtrum, obliquely set eyes and low set ears have all been described. Also, some children with HIV encephalopathy develop microcephaly.

Definition of HIV infection for infants and children under 15 months

1 Virus in blood or tissues*.
2 HIV antibody plus evidence of both cellular and humeral immune deficiency plus one or more categories in Class P2 (see above).
3 Symptoms and signs meeting the CDC case definition for AIDS.

* This should probably now include detection of HIV *antigen.*

Classification of HIV infection in children under 13 years

As many very sick children with HIV infection do not fit the CDC definition of AIDS the acronym is used less often for children. Their disease classification broadly separates infected children into two groups – symptomatic and asymptomatic. There are separate subclasses and categories to include LIP and recurrent serious bacterial infections (category PO includes perinatally exposed infants and children up to *15 months* of age who are HIV antibody positive but who cannot be classified as definitely infected).

Part 3 Other sexually transmitted diseases in HIV positive patients

When following HIV positive patients it is important to monitor for other sexually transmitted diseases. Interestingly, in this group syphilis may be missed as the VDRL can be negative or in low titre (see **254**). Otherwise the manifestations of syphilis are no different from the usual. It seems that this group of patients is particularly vulnerable to herpes simplex. Hepatitis B seems not to be unusually severe. However, hepatitis B vaccination should probably be given to all HIV positive patients at risk. Antibody response to the vaccine may be impaired.

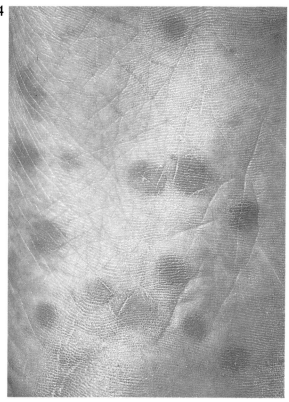

254 **Secondary syphilis** in a patient with AIDS. This patient with florid secondary syphilis had a VDRL titre of only 1:2.

Part 4   Counselling of patients with HIV disease

No book on AIDS would be complete without discussion of the psychological as well as the strictly medical needs of the patients.

Few diseases are as frightening to patients as AIDS and yet, as well as the fear of death, they often have to face a cruel rejection by their friends and society. Many homosexual patients may develop AIDS or ARC before they have come to terms with their own homosexuality and they must also face up to this and work through feelings of guilt that may cause them to suffer even more.

It is important, if patients are going to be able to cope, that their doctors talk openly and honestly to them about their condition and, if appropriate, about their guilt and the fact that they might be dying. The greatest complaint from patients is that they are not told enough about their disease – in fact the situation can even arise when the patients know more about it than their doctors. They want to know so much about what they can do to help themselves, how they can prevent transmitting the disease to others and what treatments are available to them – and they should be given time to discuss these matters. A detailed handout is a useful adjunct – it enables the patient to review the facts outside the doctor's office where stress means that much of what is said is forgotten.

Counselling is particularly important when it comes to the use of the HIV antibody test. It is vital if this test is to be performed on relatively well patients that they understand this is a test which indicates the likely presence of the AIDS virus, and that a positive result does not in itself mean AIDS. Except in unusual circumstances this test should not be performed without the knowledge and consent of the patient and the result should be treated in the strictest confidence. A patient receiving a positive result may require considerable counselling and certainly deserves detailed information. The physician may often have to prescribe for symptoms of the hyperventilation syndrome and irritable bowel syndrome, so marked is the anxiety. The best treatment for these however, is probably a sympathetic ear and a promise of support.

Part 5   Transmission and prevention of HIV disease

The principal means of transmission of HIV infection are anal and/or vaginal intercourse and the sharing of intravenous needles and 'gear' by drug addicts. Blood and blood product transfusion did account for some 2% of cases early in the epidemic; however, the screening of blood donations with HIV antibody test, and the heat treatment of factor VIII, have essentially eliminated these modes of transmission. Other forms of sexual activity such as oral sex, although possible routes of transmission, appear to carry considerably less risk.

It would appear that trauma in sexual intercourse is not required for the transmission of the virus, as artificial insemination of semen alone has been responsible for infection in humans and other primates.

The risk of transmission of HIV to health workers appears to be extremely low. The only significant risk seems to be needle stick injury. Less than 0.5% of needle stick injuries involving HIV antibody positive patients and seronegative health workers however have resulted in seroconversion in the health worker. This suggests the virus is less infectious in this route than hepatitis B. Needle stick injury from an HBeAg positive carrier results in about a 17% conversion rate in seronegative individuals. Although the risk for health workers is small, great care should be taken whenever sharps are involved. Needles should be immediately discarded into a sharps bin without resheathing, or removal from the syringe, unless some form of extra protection device such as a 'needle guard' is attached to the sheath (257). Needles should not be left for others to clear up.

Other precautions that should be taken are always to ensure that the patient is lying down for venipuncture to avoid syncope, and to have the sharps bin close to hand. A vacuvenous system rather than a syringe is recommended wherever possible as it excludes the possibility of injection of fluids following a needle prick injury. Gloves should be worn whenever dealing with body fluids, and spill should be mopped up using sodium hypochlorite (259) as a disinfectant. If it is a surface on which bleach cannot be used, hot soapy water will suffice.

255   The hazards of trying to resheath a needle. Resheathing should never be performed in this way.

During all operative procedures the only additional precaution to the usual gloves, gowns and masks that should be used is eye protection. Instruments are adequately sterilized by heat. Instruments that cannot be subjected to heat are best sterilized using glutaraldehyde which renders HIV harmless very quickly. A half hour submersion is recommended although the virus is probably rendered inactive within seconds. Sodium hypochlorite should not be used to sterilise instruments as it causes them to rust.

256 Venepuncture in a patient with AIDS. Note the precautions: patient lying down to prevent syncopy, sharps bin close to operator, Vacutainer usage, operator wearing gloves.

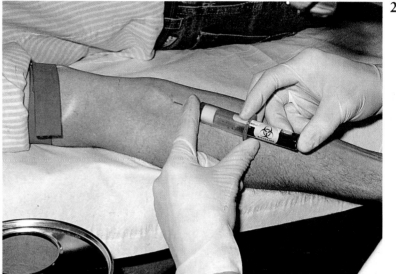

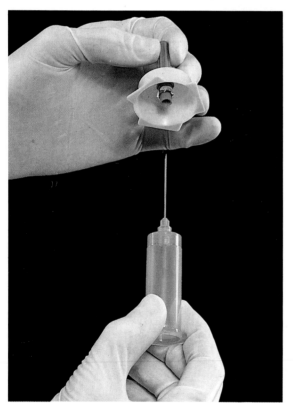

257 Disposal of needle with safety guard.

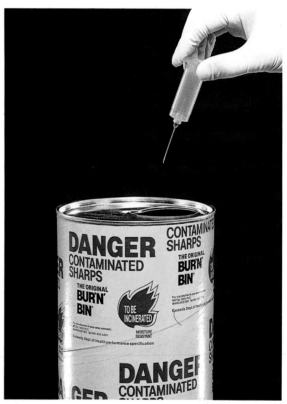

258 Sharps bin.

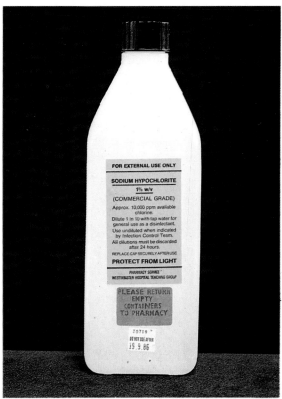

259 Hypochlorite for mopping up spilled blood.

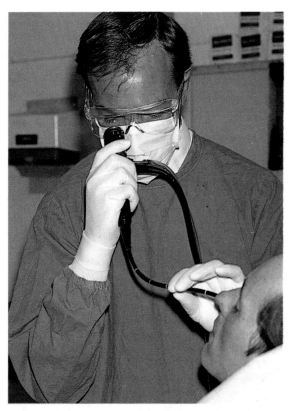

260 Fibreoptic bronchoscopy being performed with operator wearing eye protection.

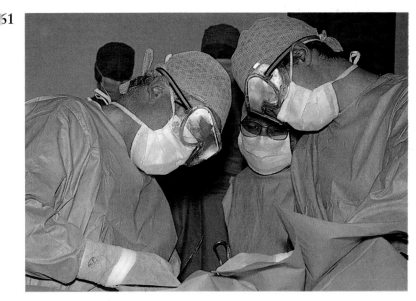

261 Lymph node biopsy being performed. Surgeons wearing eye protection.

Special precautions in the dental surgery

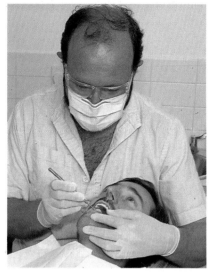

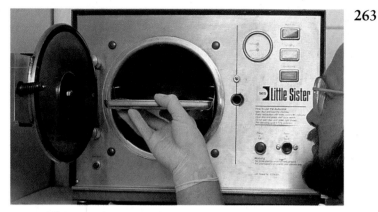

263   All instruments autoclaved.

262   Dentist wearing gloves, mask and eye protection.

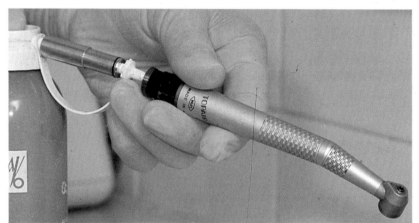

264   Sterilisation for a dental handpiece.

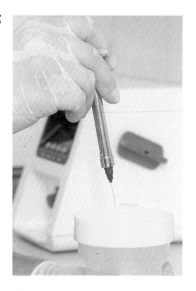

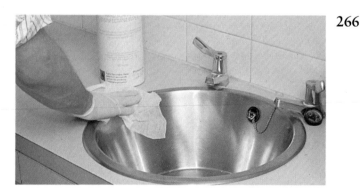

266   Special cleaning of surfaces in the surgery with viricidal disinfectant.

265   All sharps carefully disposed of in sharps bins. This model is a special one to grasp the needle of the dental syringe for unscrewing.

Now that the hepatitis B virus and HIV are widespread it is essential that dentists institute good infection control procedures in order to protect themselves and their patients. The precautions need not be excessive but must be applied to every patient, as only a minority of patients will be aware if they carry HIV and even if aware a patient may not inform his dentist.

1 Gloves should always be used when touching blood, saliva or mucous membranes. They should be changed between patients and hands should be washed.

2 Surgical masks and protective eyewear should be worn if blood or saliva could be spattered. (**262**).

3 Disposable gowns or washable work overalls or shirts should be worn. Gowns or work clothing should be changed daily or when soiled with blood.

4 Instruments which come into contact with oral tissue should be sterilised after use. Debris should be removed by scrubbing with soap and water before sterilisation. Instruments should be sterilised by autoclaving, i.e. the use of steam under pressure (**263**). Three minutes sterilisation at 134°C is an adequate minimum. Dry heat takes longer – two hours at 150°C-160°C. Heat sensitive instruments may be sterilised using glutaraldehyde.

The dental handpiece: handpieces should also be sterilised between patients. Many can now be autoclaved after lubricating with the correct oil. A good supply of handpieces will avoid delays because of sterilisation procedures. If a handpiece cannot be sterilised it should be flushed through with water or a sterilising spray (**263**), wrapped in paper towelling soaked in glutaraldehyde, placed in a sealed plastic bag and left for 10 minutes. Before use it should be rinsed again with water.

5 Surfaces should be decontaminated by wiping down with sodium hypochlorite or an iodophor (**265**). Surfaces difficult to disinfect should be isolated with an impervious cover, e.g. plastic.

6 Droplet and aerosol production should be avoided where possible by use of rubber dams and high speed evacuation.

7 Great care should be taken with hypodermic needles and a sharps bin is essential (see above). Special sharps containers are available for use with dental syringes which enable the needle to be unscrewed from the syringe without resheathing (**264**).

Abbreviations

AIDS – Acquired immunodeficiency syndrome

ARC – AIDS-related complex

CMV – Cytomegalovirus

CDC – Center for Disease Control

EBV – Epstein-Barr virus

ELISA – Enzyme-linked immunosorbent assay

H & E – Haematoxylin and cosin

HIV – Human immunodeficiency virus

LAV – Lymphadenopathy-associated virus

PCP – Pneumocystis carinii pneumonia

PGL – Persistent generalised lymphadenopathy

RIPA – Radio-immune precipitin assay

XLD – Xylose Lysine Desoxycholate agar

Appendix A

The full definition of AIDS

(CDC Sept. 1987)

A case of AIDS is defined as an illness characterized by one or more of the following "indicator" diseases, depending on the status of laboratory evidence for HIV infection:

I. Without laboratory evidence regarding HIV infection:

If laboratory tests for HIV were not performed or gave indeterminate results, any of the conditions in the list below would indicate AIDS if it was diagnosed by a **definitive** method and the patient had none of the other causes of immunodeficiency listed below that could explain the occurrence of the indicator disease:

1   *Pneumocystis carinii* pneumonia.

2   Toxoplasmosis of the brain in a patient >1 month of age.

3   Cryptosporidiosis with diarrhoea persisting for >1 month.

4   Candidiasis of the oesphagus, trachea, bronchi or lungs.

5   Extrapulmonary cryptococcosis.

6   *Mycobacterium avium* complex or *M. kansasii* disease at a site other than lungs or lymph nodes.

7   Cytomegalovirus infection of an internal organ other than liver in a patient >1 month of age.

8   Herpes simplex virus infection causing a mucocutaneous ulcer that persists for more than 1 month, or bronchitis, pneumonitis, or oesophagitis for any duration in a patient >1 month of age.

9   Progressive multifocal leucoencephalopathy.

10   Primary lymphoma of the brain in a patient <60 years of age.

11   Kaposi's sarcoma in a patient <60 years of age.

12   PLH/LIP complex (pulmonary lymphoid hyperplasia and/or lymphoid interstitial pneumonia) in a child <13 years of age.

Causes of immunodeficiency that disqualify diseases as indicators of AIDS in the absence of antibody evidence for HIV infection:

a.   High-dose or long-term systemic corticosteroid therapy or other immunosuppressive/cytotoxic therapy within three months before the onset of the indicator disease.

b.   Hodgkin's disease, non-Hodgkin's lymphoma (other than primary brain lymphoma), lymphocytic leukaemia, multiple myeloma, or another cancer of lymphoreticular or histiocytic tissue, or angioimmunoblastic lymphadenopathy, diagnosed before or within three months after diagnosis of the indicator disease.

c.   A genetic (congenital) immunodeficiency syndrome or an acquired immunodeficiency syndrome atypical of HIV infection, such as one involving hypogammaglobulinaemia.

II. With laboratory evidence for HIV infection:

In the presence of antibody evidence for HIV infection.

Any of the conditions listed above or below indicates AIDS regardless of the presence of other causes of immunodeficiency:

A. Diseases diagnosed definitively

13   Isosporiasis with diarrhoea persisting >1 month.

14   Extrapulmonary or disseminated histoplasmosis.

15   Extrapulmonary or disseminated coccidio·idomycosis.

16   Extrapulmonary or disseminated tuberculosis.

17   Any noncutaneous extrapulmonary or disseminated mycobacterial infection other than tuberculosis or leprosy.

18   Recurrent non-typhoid *Salmonella* septicaemia.

19   Multiple or recurrent bacterial infections (any combination of >2 within a two year period) of the following types in a child <13 years of age:

   septicaemia, pneumonia, meningitis, bone or joint infection, or abscess of an internal organ or body cavity (excluding otitis media or superficial skin or mucosal abscesses), caused by *Haemophilus*, *Streptococcus* (including pneumococcus), or other pyogenic bacteria.

20   Kaposi's sarcoma at any age.

21   Primary lymphoma of the brain at any age.

22   Other non-Hodgkin's lymphoma of B-cell immunologic phenotype:

   small noncleaved lymphoma (Burkitt's tumour or Burkitt-like lymphoma)
   or
   immunoblastic sarcoma (large cell lymphoma, diffuse histiocytic lymphoma, diffuse undifferentiated lymphoma, reticulum cell sarcoma, or high-grade lymphoma).

Note: Lymphomas are not included if they are of T-cell immunological phenotype or are described as "lymphocytic", "lymphoblastic", "small cleaved" or "plasmacytoid lymphocytic".

23   HIV encephalopathy ("AIDS demential complex")*.

24   HIV wasting syndrome ("slim disease")**.

B.   Diseases diagnosed presumptively

● *Pneumocystis carinii* pneumonia.

● Toxoplasmosis of the brain in a patient >1 month of age.

● Oesophageal candidiasis.

● Extrapulmonary or disseminated mycobacterial infection (acid-fast bacilli of undetermined species).

● Kaposi's sarcoma.

● Lymphoid interstitial pneumonitis (LIP/PLH complex) in a child <13 years of age.

*HIV encepalopathy:
   Clinical findings of disabling cognitive and/or motor dysfunction interfering with occupation or activities of daily living, or loss of behavioural developmental milestones in a child, progressing over weeks to months, in the absence of a concurrent illness or condition other than HIV infection that could explain the findings. Methods to rule out such concurrent illnesses and conditions must include cerebrospinal fluid examination and either brain imaging (computed tomography or magnetic resonance) or autopsy.

**HIV wasting syndrome:
   Findings of profound involuntary weight loss (more than 10% of baseline body weight) plus other chronic diarrhoea (lasting >1 month) or documented chronic fever and weakness (lasting >1 month) in the absence of a concurrent illness or condition other than HIV infection that could explain the findings (e.g. cancer, tuberculosis, cryptosporidiosis or other specific enteritis).

III.   With evidence against HIV infection:

With laboratory test results negative for HIV infection, AIDS is ruled out for surveillance purposes unless the patient has had:

1.   Either of the following:

● *Pneumocystis carinii* pneumonia diagnosed by a definitive method, or
● a. any of the other diseases indicative of AIDS listed above in Section 1 diagnosed by a definitive method, and
   b.   a T-helper (T4) lymphocyte count <400 per mm^3.

2.   None of the other causes of immunodeficiency listed above in Section 1.

Reference. MMWR 1987;36(suppl no 15):35-155.

Appendix B

AIDS in Africa

By M. Rolfe, MRCP, DTM&H

HIV infection and AIDS are now endemic throughout most of Central and East Africa. The magnitude of the problem facing many countries is considerable but precise data is often lacking as diagnostic facilities are limited and under-reporting common. It is still predominantly an urban disease but is beginning to spread into the rural areas.

Infection in Africa is spread in three main ways; by heterosexual intercourse, by vertical transplacental transmission from mother to child and by blood transfusion. Homosexuality is rare in Africa and intravenous drug abuse does not occur. The role played by the use of contaminated needles and instruments is unknown but is unlikely to be significant.

HIV infection produces a wide spectrum of clinical disease in Africa and there are some significant differences from the developed world. Pneumocystis carinii pneumonia seems much less frequent even allowing for the lack of sophisticated diagnostic equipment. Tuberculosis however, is commonly associated with HIV infection, around 40% of patients being seropositive. Although classical disease is common, the presentation may be atypical. Relapse, especially after short course chemotherapy, may occur thus adding to the cost of treatment. Drug reactions may complicate management. Tuberculous lymphadenitis may be absent in seropositive patients. Atypical mycobacterial infections also occur but data is lacking.

Enteropathic AIDS, or slim disease as it is known in Uganda, affects substantial numbers of African patients with devastating results. Chronic watery diarrhoea, which may be choleraic, with fevers and colicky abdominal pain produces malabsorption and cachexia. It is multifactorial in origin; Cryptosporidium, Isospora belli, atypical mycobacteria and Candida may all play a part. There is presently no effective treatment.

Mucocutaneous disease also appears to be more common in African patients. Many patients develop a non-specific papular rash which is intensely pruritic. Eczema, seborrhoeic dermatitis, psoriasis and alopecia also occur. Sometimes the hair loses its typical African appearance and becomes soft and straight. The presence of oral or oesophageal candidiasis indicates a poor prognosis. Oral hairy leukoplakia does not seem to occur in Africans; it may be associated with a homosexual life-style.

Herpes zoster is a strong marker of seropositivity in Africa, around 90% of all patients being seropositive. It seems to occur early in the illness, commonly involves several dermatomes, often in the head or neck and may be recurrent. Post-herpetic neuralgia seems rare probably because these patients are generally younger. Generalised herpes zoster might be expected to occur more frequently in immunocompromised patients; this does not seem to be the case although the reasons are not understood.

Kaposi's sarcoma (KS) affects some 5% of seropositive patients in Africa as opposed to 25-30% in America. Although there has been some increase in the number of patients with classical endemic KS the main change has been the appearance of a more aggressive atypical form of the disease which runs a more rapid fulminating course. The typical skin nodules appear black, rather than mauve or purple, on the African skin. Deposits may be found on the palate, gums or conjuctiva. Generalised lymphadenopathy may occur which may be discrete or massive. Involvement of the bronchial mucosa may lead to chest signs and infiltrations on chest x-ray while pleural or pericardial effusions may occur. Gastrointestinal involvement seems common but is rarely symptomatic.

Generalised lymphadenopathy is common and may occur at unusual sites such as the posterior occipital, deep cervical or submental regions. Enlargement of the epitrochlear node may be an important physical sign of HIV infection in Africans. Gland biopsy may occasionally be required to exclude tuberculosis or Kaposi's sarcoma. Neurological syndromes such as AIDS-dementia complex, myelopathy or peripheral neuropathy all occur although precise data is lacking. Toxoplasma encephalitis may be common although under-diagnosed. Cryptococcal meningitis occurs but is rarely treatable.

The true incidence of paediatric AIDS in Africa is unknown but is likely to be considerable. Serological screening is not performed at antenatal clinics to allow counselling, and around 50% of babies born to seropositive mothers will themselves develop the disease. Progression to full-blown AIDS probably develops more rapidly in children than adults.

Failure to thrive is a common presentation with repeated infections, fevers and diarrhoea leading to frank protein-calorie malnutrition. Lymphadenopathy, pneumonia, oral monilia and anaemia are all common. Part of the examination of the sick child should include an examination of the mother for lymphadenopathy, oral monilia, Kaposi's sarcoma and scars of herpes zoster.

There has been concern regarding the use of live vaccines; at the present time the benefits are thought to outweigh the potential risks. It is not known whether malaria occurs more frequently in seropositive children. Kaposi's sarcoma is now occurring in children. It usually presents with lymphadenopathy which may be massive. Biopsy is required for diagnosis as skin and oral lesions are unusual. Some children contract HIV infection through blood transfusion. At special risk are those with sickle cell anaemia or anaemia following malaria.

HIV infection has added a huge additional burden to the health services of many African countries; a lack of money, resources and trained personnel has impeded efforts to control spread of the infection. In the absence of a cure or vaccine, prevention can only be achieved through education. Unfortunately modern mass media techniques are not appropriate in Africa, and new educational approaches will have to be adapted to the various African cultures.

A1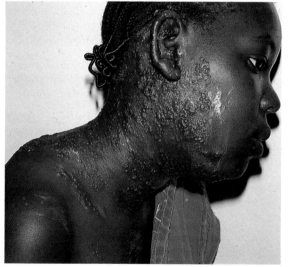

A2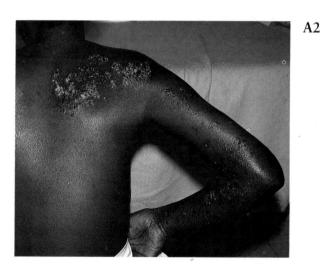

A1 Extensive herpes zoster of C2-3 in an 18-year-old girl.

A2 Herpes zoster affecting C4-6 in a 20-year-old girl.

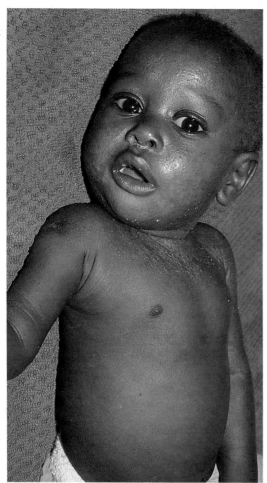

A3

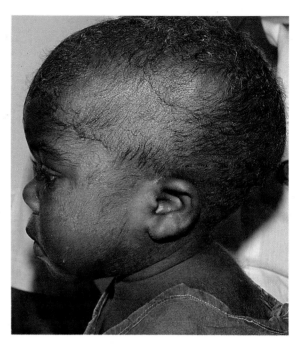

A4

A3 Six-month-old boy with disseminated BCG infection. Note BCG scar on right shoulder and eczematous rash around the neck. Glands in the right axilla were markedly enlarged and he also had generalised lymphadenopathy, splenomegaly and fever. He responded to anti-tuberculous treatment.

A4 18-month-old boy with peculiar hair distribution on forehead and cheeks. It has lost its typical African appearance and become soft and downy. Mother was HIV positive.

A5

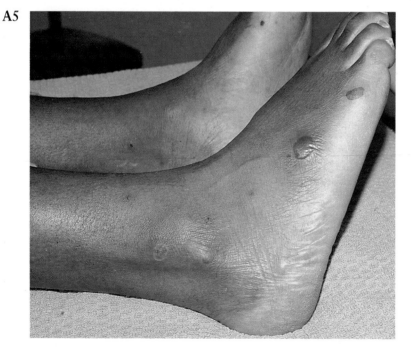

A5 Vasculitis in a 45-year-old man. Haemorrhagic blisters developed on the hands and feet together with swelling of wrists. Cleared spontaneously in two weeks.

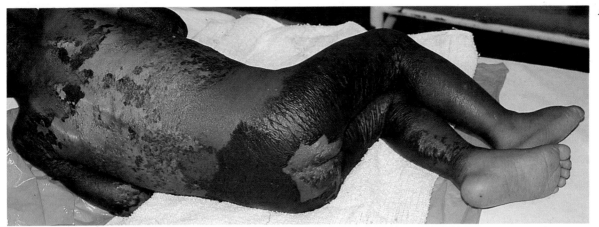

A6 Two-year-old girl with severe marasmic-kwashiorkor. Note ankle oedema and extensive desquamating hyper-pigmented rash. Child presented initially with miliary tuberculosis. Both parents seropositive.

A7 Tuberculous lymphadenitis in a 2-year-old boy.

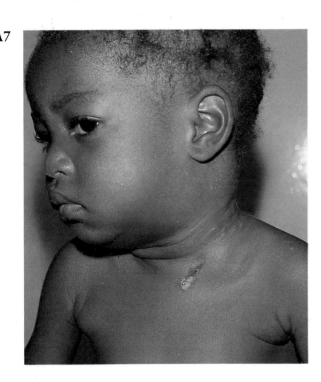

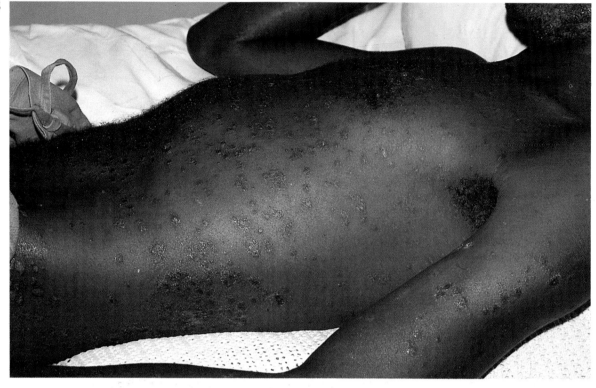

A8 Acute generalised psoriatic rash in a 35-year-old man.

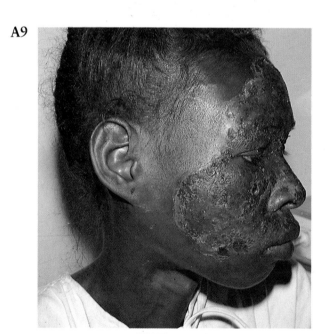

A9 Butterfly rash suggestive of discoid lupus in a 22-year-old girl. Biopsy showed non-specific changes. Responded to chloroquine. Note hair which has become soft and straight.

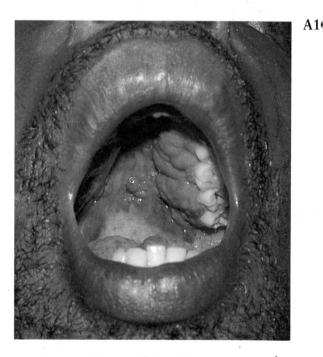

A10 Typical lesions of Kaposi's sarcoma on palate and gums in a 19-year-old man.

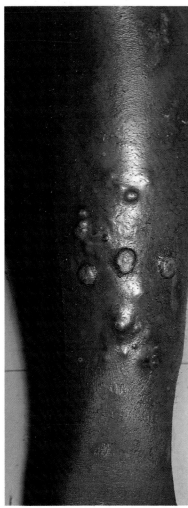

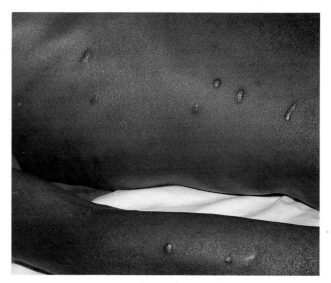

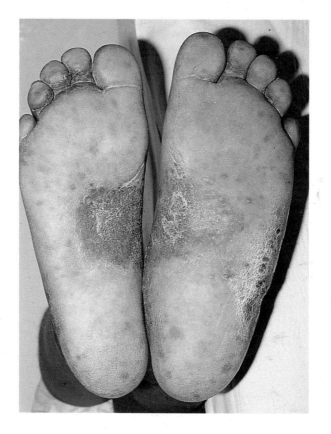

A11 Ulcerating nodules of Kaposi's sarcoma on the leg of a 25-year-old man.

A12 Typical skin lesions of Kaposi's sarcoma.

A13 Symmetrical plaques of Kaposi's sarcoma involving the soles of the feet.

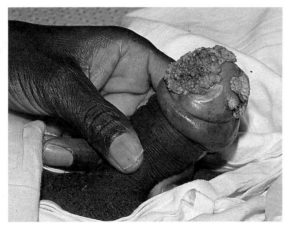

A14 Papilliferous tumours on glans penis in a man with Kaposi's sarcoma.

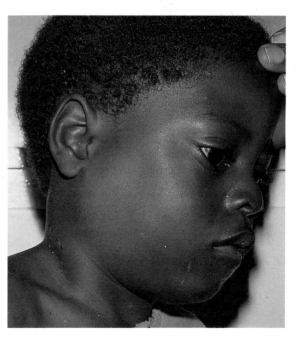

A15 Lymphadenopathy in a 5-year-old boy. Biopsy showed Kaposi's sarcoma. Skin and oral lesions are unusual in children. There were fluffy shadows on chest x-ray suggesting lung involvement. No history of blood transfusion but both parents were seropositive.

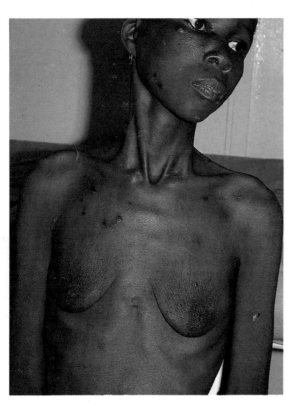

A16 Skin lesions of Kaposi's sarcoma in a 21-year-old woman. Note nodules on the face and wasted appearance.

Appendix C

Treatment options in Kaposi's sarcoma

Radiotherapy

Kaposi's sarcoma is almost invariably sensitive to radiotherapy and this is the treatment of choice for any large plaque. Lesions on the shins or on the soles of the feet are best treated early; if left untreated they usually cause ankle oedema or pain. Radiotherapy usually results in the arrest of further growth and flattening of lesions – haemosiderin stain the same size as the lesion often remains, however. This is another reason for treating early – especially for lesions on the face.

Lesions in the mouth should generally not be treated with radiotherapy as the patients are likely to suffer severely from ulceration of the oral mucosa, 'mucositis', as a side effect (**193**, page 70). Patients with HIV disease seem much more sensitive to this particular side effect of radiotherapy. When there are multiple small lesions scattered over the body, electron beam radiotherapy, if available, is more practical than conventional radiotherapy.

Lesions may sometimes reactivate after initial flattening with radiotherapy.

Intralesional chemotherapy

When lesions are very small (less than 1 cm in diameter) and not too numerous, intralesional injection of 0.1 to 0.2ml of vinblastine (0.2 mg/ml) will often arrest growth of and sometimes totally eradicate them (**194**, **195**, page 71). Initially there is a minor inflammatory reaction which soon settles. Some lesions need to be treated more than once.

This is a particularly useful treatment to stop the growth of small lesions on the face before they become unsightly. It can be performed in the surgery and is more convenient than radiotherapy which might, for example, be difficult to justify for two or three lesions of 0.5cm diameter. It is probably best avoided for

nasal lesions when early radiotherapy is very useful to prevent the development of an unsightly blue nose (**176** to **179**, page 67).

Systemic chemotherapy

When lesions are widespread and multiple or there is gingival or visceral involvement systemic chemotherapy is justified. The decision to begin therapy is not based simply on the extent of disease but also on the rate of development of new lesions. There is the possibility that chemotherapy may further immuno-compromise an already immunocompromised individual, worsening the prognosis through increased susceptibility to opportunistic infection. Although control studies have not been performed it is probably fair to say that with single agent chemotherapy such as bleomycin, vincristine, vinblastine and Etoposide (VP16), this is not true to any significant degree. Patients have not suddenly acquired more infections when treated with these agents. Deterioration has, however, been noted with adriamycin, which causes depression of cell mediated immunity and should be avoided in these immunocompromised patients.

Systemic chemotherapy is normally administered to AIDS Kaposi patients for cosmetic reasons or for the relief of pain or oedema. As many Kaposi patients die from infection rather than from a tumour the expectation is not that life will necessarily be prolonged by the treatment. In cases of aggressive tumours however, especially those involving the lungs, single agent or combination systemic chemotherapy will sometimes prolong life (**198**, **199**, page 72).

The choice of chemotherapy will depend on circumstances – with many patients now being treated with AZT (zidovudine, Retrovir) marrow-sparing agents such as bleomycin and vincristine are used more frequently than vinblastine or VP16.

Appendix D

Advice for people who are HIV antibody positive

Individuals who have a positive HIV antibody test have at some stage been infected with HIV (The Human Immunodeficiency Virus – formerly known as HTLV-III/LAV). This virus has recently been discovered to be the cause of AIDS but it is not known what percentage of infected individuals will go on to develop AIDS. To date only a minority have done so.

Most infected individuals however do appear to be carriers of HIV and to remain infectious. The presence of antibodies in the blood does not mean, as it does with some other infections, that the virus has left the body and the individual is immune.

The commonest way HIV causes illness in an individual, if it is going to do so, is by lowering the body's resistance to infectious disease i.e. damaging the body's 'immune system'. It does this by infecting a certain subset of one of the types of white blood cell. All white blood cells are concerned with defence against infection (i.e. they are part of the body's immune system) but it is a certain subset of the lymphocytes that HIV infects. Lymphocytes are particularly concerned with defence against viral, fungal and parasitic infection and some types of tumour. The particular subset of the lymphocyte population that gets infected is the 'T helper lymphocytes' – sometimes referred to as the 'OKT4 positive or CD4 positive lymphocytes'. These T helper cells are an important component of the immune system and if their function is reduced or their numbers significantly depleted by HIV, defects in cell-mediated immunity develop which may result in the development of major or minor opportunistic infections or tumours.

Individuals who have been infected with HIV can be divided into four general groups:

1 Well with no signs of infection or immunosuppression. Such individuals could be called asymptomatic carriers.

2 Well with glandular swellings (lymphadenopathy) in armpits, neck, etc. Such individuals are said to have persistent generalised lymphadenopathy (PGL).

3 Less than well with fatigue, often night sweats, and often a low T Helper lymphocyte subset count.

Such individuals have minor infections such as shingles or oral thrush which indicate a degree of immunosuppression. These individuals have been classified as having AIDS related complex (ARC).

4 Individuals who meet the Centre for Disease Control's (CDC) criteria for the acquired immune deficiency syndrome (AIDS).

To meet this definition the individual must have Kaposi's sarcoma or have had a life-threatening opportunistic infection such as pneumocystis pneumonia or toxoplasmosis. Such individuals nearly always have a low T helper lymphocyte count.

Although one can only state with certainty that individuals in category three and four are immunocompromised it is often true that those in categories one and two are also immunocompromised to some degree. The T helper lymphocyte count whilst a useful guide to immune status only measures the number of CD4 positive cells and not their function and thus should not be relied upon too heavily. Anyone who is HIV antibody positive should therefore regard himself as possibly immunocompromised and take note of the following health guidelines.

Report early

If you are immunocompromised and you develop an infection it is best to report early to the physician who cares for your HIV disease for assessment and for an antibiotic if necessary. This is standard advice given to any group of immunocompromised patients, e.g. kidney transplant recipients, as infections may develop more quickly and be more severe in any immunocompromised individual.

Having said this however, an individual immunocompromised from HIV infection is not at risk of dying from the common cold and minor infections are more common than major ones. Identifying that you have an infection is usually not difficult, but signs of infection do very much depend on the site of that infection – cough and breathlessness usually means a chest infection, diarrhoea a bowel infection, a rash possibly a skin infection, etc. Infection is often accompanied by fever.

An increased swelling of your lymph glands usually does not mean an acute infection. It is usual for glands to swell intermittently in individuals with PGL, particularly if you get over-tired, and you should not be alarmed by this – if anything it may be reassuring in as much as it indicates activity in the immune system. Rest if your glands swell. If any particular gland is persistently enlarging however, show it to your doctor.

Rest

Fatigue is the commonest symptom experienced by individuals with HIV infection. The fatigue may come and go with patients feeling quite well for variable periods of time and then experiencing periods of severe fatigue with loss of energy, loss of ambition and drowsiness. It is often difficult however to separate true fatigue from the lassitude that accompanies depression.

The fatigue should be acknowledged and patients should rest as much as possible. We recommend at least 8 hours of sleep each night and short naps during those periods when the fatigue is profound. If fatigue is so severe that you have difficulty in completing a day's work, a week or two of sick leave with ample rest is certainly appropriate.

This recommendation may require a major change in your social life. If you are accustomed to going out at the weekend, staying up late, spending time with friends at a bar, or dancing until the early hours of the morning these behaviour patterns need to be recognised and altered. You should attempt to see friends for small dinners or evenings in the theatre or cinema. You should decide which hour each night you will be in bed, and your friends must be made aware that your health is the most important thing in your life, and that you are going to stick to your schedule of getting to bed by 10 or 11 each evening. Of paramount importance is that you should listen to your body and if you feel that you should rest, that should be the course of action to follow.

Exercise

Regular exercise is desirable but to overdo it is tiring and unwise. If you attend a gym it is probably best to continue but not to necessarily step up your programme – exercise to keep fit but not to exhaustion. If you have not been in the habit of exercising you should begin slowly – perhaps with regular walking or swimming. We advise against competitive sports because in the heat of competition an individual may push himself harder than he should.

Diet

A balanced diet with a reasonable calorie and fibre content is recommended. Potatoes and rice are good sources of carbohydrate. Beans, cheese and meat are high in protein. Vegetables and fruit are high in fibre. You may consider adding bran to your diet for further fibre.

There is no need to go on any 'special' diet however.

Vitamins

If your diet is adequate in greens and fruit, vitamin supplementation is usually unnecessary. Some signs of HIV infection however may mimic Vitamin C and zinc deficiency, so occasionally we recommend to some patients that they take Vitamin C or zinc tablets.

Drugs

Alcohol in moderation (2 drinks per day) does not appear to have any adverse effect. The most common opportunistic infection experienced by people with HIV is however pneumocystis pneumonia – a chest infection. Smoking cigarettes will irritate your lungs, and theoretically could increase your chance of pneumocystis infection. Patients are urged to stop smoking cigarettes. Other recreational drugs are probably also unwise – especially stimulant drugs (cocaine, speed, poppers) as they give a false sense of 'energy' which when used leaves the body exhausted. Moderation is probably the key word.

Sex

Individuals infected with HIV are capable of transmitting this agent to their sexual partners before they develop any symptoms whatsoever.

Exactly which sexual activities transmit the virus and which do not is unknown. However, surveys of gay men who restrict themselves to only certain practices give us an indication of relative risk.

Homosexual men who have been mainly passive in anal intercourse are much more likely than others to be HIV antibody positive. Male homosexuals who have restricted themselves exclusively to active anal intercourse or oral sex are far less likely to be HIV antibody positive. It is impossible to prove however that any particular sexual practice is safe and there are now many HIV positive male homosexuals who insist they have never had passive anal intercourse and many HIV antibody positive heterosexual men who have contracted the infection by vaginal intercourse with infected women. There are few, if any, male homosexuals who have restricted themselves only to oral sex, who are HIV antibody positive.

What, therefore, are the guidelines on sexual practice for HIV antibody positive patients? Different doctors will give different advice but we feel it is important to remember that if, as an HIV antibody positive individual, you have unprotected vaginal or anal intercourse (active or passive) with an individual who is HIV antibody negative or whose status is unknown, you are very likely to transmit the AIDS virus.

Remember also that a condom, while a good protection if it remains intact, may break (especially with anal intercourse), and if it does is no protection at all. It would seem wise therefore for HIV antibody positive men to cease altogether active anal or vaginal intercourse with partners who are HIV antibody negative or who do not know their status.

What of other sexual practices with HIV antibody negative individuals? The only way of being absolutely certain of not transmitting infection is to have entirely 'non-mucous membrane' contact or 'dry' sex. However as mentioned above oral sex appears to be low risk. Passive vaginal or anal sex on the part of an HIV antibody positive female (or passive homosexual men) with the active negative partner wearing a condom continuously is also probably low risk. Kissing must be very low risk, if a risk at all, as nearly all cases of HIV infection have had actual intercourse or received blood and one would expect many unexplained cases of kissing alone could transmit the virus. Although live virus has been isolated from saliva and therefore theoretically considerable saliva exchange could transmit the virus, no cases of such transmission have been clearly documented.

What about sex with other HIV antibody positive individuals? Here medical opinion is again divided. Arguments against having sex with other patients are that you may pick up another strain of HIV worse than your own or you may pick up another infection such as syphilis which may further damage the immune system or trigger dormant HIV infection. Another worry regarding anal sex is that sperm in the rectum if absorbed into the blood may itself be immunosuppressive. These worries, though logical, are theoretical. It would seem wise however if you do intend having anal or vaginal sex with other HIV antibody positive individuals to use condoms. If you do intend to use condoms buy a generous supply and use plenty of *water-based* lubricant to prevent tearing from friction. Do not use saliva or oil-based lubricants. Saliva may contain the virus and oils penetrate the latex of condoms causing them to split. We recommend using water-based gels which contain nonoxinol – a spermicidal agent which destroys HIV.

Ultimately the decision about whom to have sex with and what practices to indulge in is of course a personal one. Restricting anal or vaginal sex only to an already regular partner or partners whom you know to be positive, using condoms, and having only 'safer', or entirely safe dry sex with antibody negative individuals is what most antibody positive individuals decide. Obviously it is vital not to transmit this infection to those who are not already infected or to do anything that would further impair your own immunity.

Social activities

It is now common knowledge that an HIV antibody positive individual is not an infective risk to others in an ordinary social or family setting. The only advice we would give is that an HIV antibody positive individual should not share a toothbrush or razor blade with others as these objects allow the possibility of blood contact. Sharing glasses and knives and forks is probably not a good practice for anyone to indulge in but is very unlikely to transmit HIV if it occurred accidentally. Dishes should be washed in hot soapy water but no other special precaution is necessary. Soiled linen only requires to be laundered in a hot wash. Blood or other body fluid spills should be mopped up using household bleach as an anti-virus disinfectant (one in ten dilution). On surfaces that may be damaged by bleach hot soapy water will suffice.

There is no reason for an HIV antibody positive individual to avoid social contact for the protection of his own health. We know of no situation where immunocompromised people have suddenly developed pneumocystis or other opportunistic infections from being exposed to individuals suffering from these diseases. It would appear that nearly all of us already carry many opportunistic organisms such as Pneumocystis carini and Cytomegalovirus (CMV). What determines whether we become ill from them or not is the state of our immune system and not whether we are re-exposed to these agents.

Blood/organ donation

No HIV antibody positive individual should carry an organ donor card or donate blood to the blood transfusion service. This in fact applies to all gay men and intravenous drug users whether HIV antibody positive or not.

Vaccinations

Although they have not yet proved to be harmful, HIV antibody positive individuals should probably not receive live vaccines such as those for polio or yellow fever. All inactivated (dead) vaccines such as Hep B Vac and 'flu vaccine' must be safe however.

Treatment

Nearly all the opportunistic infections acquired secondary to immunosuppression are treatable, but there is a greater chance of success if treatment is commenced early.

There are also various treatments available for the underlying immunosuppression itself. Such treatments are of two kinds 'immunostimulant' drugs which to date have shown only slight if any benefit, and 'antiviral' anti-HIV drugs, such as AZT which has been shown to improve ARC symptoms and increase survival in those patients who are able to take it longterm.

If you are offered AZT by your physician do not dismiss it lightly because of scary stories about side effects in the popular press. Its side effects are all reversible and its beneficial effect is proven. If you are unable to tolerate AZT it may be that you will be asked to partake in the assessment of other drugs. If you are, it is very important that you understand fully the possible risks and benefits and are not frightened to ask questions.

Alternative therapies

As there is at present no known cure for HIV infection and AIDs we are often asked about the benefits of alternative therapies offered by homeopathy, herbal medicine, etc. Just as there is as yet no good scientific evidence that conventional medicine can reverse AIDS neither is there any evidence that any other therapies work either. Alternative therapies are often quite harmless however and may possibly be of some benefit. If you are contemplating them ask for full information, discuss them with your doctor, and do not put your trust in literature that is not from reliable scientific source. Be especially sceptical if a large amount of money is being charged for any alternative therapy.

Support agencies

You are not alone. There are thousands of HIV antibody positive people. If you feel lonely or in need of more information and live in the United Kingdom the Terrence Higgins Trust or the Body Positive Group are two helpful organisations you can turn to. The Body Positive Group is an organisation largely made up of people who are themselves HIV antibody positive.

They may be able to help you and later you may be able to help them. If you live outside the United Kingdom ask your clinic for the names and telephone numbers of local AIDS help organisations.

Who should know?

With so much misunderstanding about HIV disease around we recommend that someone who is HIV antibody positive tells as few people as possible the result of his test. It may of course help to discuss the problem with one or two trusted friends; however if there is no one you feel you can fully trust then it may be best to talk only to people at your hospital. Do not tell your employer – he does not need to know and however understanding he may appear we have known many employers to turn nasty.

We are often asked if patients should tell their general practitioners their result. An argument against telling your GP is that he would have to include this information in any medical report you may require. However, if you are consulting your GP while unwell with unexplained symptoms then you must tell him as it might be vital to your medical care, but if you are currently quite well then there is probably no need to make a special point of telling your GP. You should inform your dentist or any doctor who is going to perform a surgical procedure. Also you should inform a tattooist, acupuncturist or ear piercer that your blood may be infectious.

The future

A question often asked by HIV antibody positive individuals is 'am I going to get AIDS?' No one can answer this question for any one individual. Hopefully many HIV antibody positive individuals will never become unwell or develop AIDS. Amongst those who are unwell with AIDS related complex a question often asked is 'does having ARC mean that I shall definitely develop AIDS?' Again no one can answer this question for any one individual either. Some patients unwell with ARC improve greatly on changing their lifestyle and taking better care of themselves and many have lived several years without developing AIDS. If you do have ARC however antiviral therapy against HIV to prevent further damage to the immune system should be considered.

Finally patients with AIDS often ask 'how long have I got to live?' No one can accurately predict how long anyone will live especially with this disease. AIDS can move quickly but can be a very slow disease. Many patients with AIDS in this country are alive and well and in full-time occupations several years after diagnosis.

Take care of yourself. Think positively. Do not transmit this infection to others. Treatments are already available and more successful ones may be just around the corner.

Index